A Spirit of Charity

First Edition Published by
Secant Publishing, LLC
P.O. Box 79
Salisbury MD 21803

ISBN: 978-1-944962-06-7 (hardcover)
ISBN: 978-1-944962-07-4 (paperback)
ISBN: 978-1-944962-08-1 (epub)
ISBN: 978-1-944962-09-8 (mobi)

Library of Congress Control Number: 2016933462

Book cover and layout design by theBookDesigners

Cover photos courtesy of: Grady Health System; Jeff Dahl, 2008,
Wikimedia Commons; Special Collections and Archives,
Georgia State University; Wikimedia Creative Commons.

A Spirit of Charity

Restoring the Bond between
America and Its Public Hospitals

Mike King

For the patients and staff at Charity Hospital,
New Orleans (1736–2005) and Grady Memorial Hospital,
Atlanta, which, thankfully, is still with us.

CONTENTS

"Better the occasional faults of a government that lives in a spirit of charity than the consistent omissions of a government frozen in the ice of its own indifference."

—FRANKLIN DELANO ROOSEVELT, *June 27, 1936*

FOREWORD

Arthur Caplan, PhD
Founding Director, Division of Medical Ethics
Drs. William F. and Virginia Connolly Mitty Professor
Department of Population Health
NYU Langone Medical Center

Two moral myths thread their way through this book. They are myths so powerful that they have long flown in the face of well-established facts. One is that America has the best health care system in the world. The other is that every American receives the same quality of care regardless of whether they are rich or poor.

These are myths that Mike King must debunk in order to explain why public charity hospitals like Grady Memorial in Atlanta, Cook County in Chicago, Jackson Memorial in Miami, Bellevue in New York City, and many others in urban areas have the mission, census, and finances that they do. If the two myths were true, a powerful argument could be made that these hospitals and others like them need not exist.

But they are just that—myths. As this book convincingly shows through its illuminating tour of both history and current affairs, our great public hospitals—the true safety nets of American health care—remain essential.

As King points out, American political leaders and physicians prominent in major medical associations often declare that America has the best health care system in the world. When, at the start of his first term, President Barack Obama proposed the Patient Protection and Affordable Care Act to

broaden access to affordable health insurance for millions of
uninsured Americans, the Republican leadership in both the
Senate and the House warned that his reform would do nothing but ruin the world's finest health care system.

It is impossible to believe that a country that had forty-one
million uninsured citizens as recently as 2013 could claim to
have the finest or best health system in the world. Even after
the Affordable Care Act was implemented in 2014, there were
still more than thirty million Americans who lacked health
insurance. No other developed nation has that large a percentage of uninsured citizens.

Those who are uninsured often cite the high cost of insurance for their lack of coverage. It is simply too expensive for
poorer people who don't qualify as poor enough for Medicaid
in their states to buy private insurance for themselves and
their families.

In 2014, many people who worked did not have access to
insurance coverage through their jobs. Poor adults in states that
did not expand their Medicaid programs—as the Affordable
Care Act encouraged states to do—remain ineligible for public coverage, even though someone would have to be absurdly
poor to gain eligibility for Medicaid in many states. In addition, there are millions of undocumented immigrants who
are ineligible for any form of insurance. People of color are at
higher risk of being uninsured than whites.

Why don't we worry about these millions of uninsured
Americans and their families? It is partly because of the Gradys.
Public hospitals take the uninsured into their ERs and handle their health crises. Because of the efforts and skill of those
who staff these public hospitals, we continue to ignore the huge
flaws and gaps in the American health care system.

The heroic administrators, health care providers, and
workforces that battle inadequate budgets and the overwhelming damage done by guns, drugs, booze, vehicular mayhem,
domestic violence, mental illness, sexual assault, premature

births, injuries to undocumented workers, gangbanging, and grueling poverty—whose work forms a core part of the focus of this book—also are a Band-Aid for a health system that is not a system but rather a patchwork of charity, debt, cost-shifting, patient diversion, waiting lists, little outreach, and poor follow-up.

The poor and those relying on programs for the poor do get care. It is care that comes late—often after asthma, high blood pressure, depression, or diabetes have done their worst. It is care that may require long hours of waiting to receive. It is care often delivered by those still in training. It is care that often is uncoordinated and thus requiring many visits, lots of bus rides, and multiple appointments. And it can be very expensive care.

Health care costs twice as much in the United States as it does anywhere else in the world with similar capabilities. The poor face more cost burden than the rich since they cannot afford the health insurance premiums these costs require, or the copays that often are charged.

"There is no such thing as a legitimate price for anything in health care," George Halvorson, former chairman of Kaiser Permanente, the giant health maintenance organization based in California, has said. Halvorson would know since his system has sought greater efficiencies for years. "Prices are made up depending on who the payer is" is the startling message he has to deliver. Even worse, surveys show Americans equate the quality of care they get with its cost.

When Medicare or the Department of Veterans Affairs or the US armed forces are paying the bills, prices tend to be lower. Private insurers bargain hard for lower prices. The uninsured, on the other hand, are stuck with the worst prices. So some hospitals drive up costs by imposing high prices on the uninsured for many services, which they try to recapture from public taxes or charity, thereby keeping their services available but not always efficiently. These hospitals are stuck in a cycle of rising cost with falling subsidies.

Maybe we could justify a much greater bill for paying for the Rube Goldberg patchwork of a health system we have if it performed much better than those in other nations. But it does not. The poor in particular often get rescued by public hospitals, but the ability of these institutions to act as front-line primary care providers seeking to prevent problems before they get started and become very expensive to manage is very low.

What about the other myth that everyone in America gets the same quality of care? In one sense that is true. When you get your gallbladder out at the Mayo Clinic, NYU Tisch, Grady, Jackson, or at Ben Taub in Houston or at Kings County in Brooklyn, everyone involved in your care is not concerned with who you are, your race, or your gender—they want to do the best job they can with the surgery. But that is where the myth ends.

You cannot and should not read this book without feeling the baleful presence of race on every page. Racism is a huge blight on American society, and its influence has driven the evolution of American health care, including the ghettoization of poor patients of color into charity hospitals. These institutions were until relatively recently segregated, underfunded, and off the attention span of middle-, upper-class, and rich Americans, with the exception of an annual charity fundraising event or two.

The Commonwealth Fund, an independent foundation, in various reports it has commissioned on health care in America, sees "Two Americas" in our health system. Who you are, where you live, and how wealthy you are play key roles, not in the quality of the care you get, but in whether you get care at all.

Looking across states, Commonwealth finds a lack of timely, affordable access to care—in particular, primary care—which undermines health, especially among low-income African-Americans and other minorities. Among low-income adults age fifty or older, fewer than half receive recommended cancer screenings and vaccines in states with greatly limited

Medicaid programs. Rates of hospital admissions for respiratory disease and the complications of diabetes are four times higher in the worst-performing Medicaid states compared with the most generous ones. For children in low-income communities, there is an eightfold spread between the highest and lowest state rates of hospitalization for asthma.

The poor who are stuck with lousy, limited Medicaid programs, mainly in the South, have double the rate of premature death before age seventy-five, infant mortality, smoking rates, obesity, and dental disease. If you get care, it is not hugely shaped or influenced by poverty or race. Whether you get any care at all before finally being wheeled into a public hospital in a crisis very much is.

Why the disparity? Racism combined with American capitalism has brought a terrible legacy in its wake. America is the only rich nation on earth that does not recognize health care as a right. We see health as something you deserve by earning it at work. If you are unemployed or underemployed but capable of full-time work, then what America offers you is mostly scorn with a bit of charity in the form of the right of entry into emergency rooms at public hospitals. These hospitals function not only under the stigma of serving the poor, often minorities or undocumented persons, but also those seen as undeserving because they did not earn their health insurance and, thus, their care.

Most nations see health care as something the community owes all of its citizens along with education and food. A few see health care as an entitlement in order to insure a competitive workforce. And some see health care as a right because it is the cheapest way to deliver care rather than using the complex bureaucracy, exclusions, copayments, and paperwork that characterize our private, employment-linked, market-based health system.

How did we get here? Why have these myths about health care lasted so long? Why is the United States the exception among our peer-nations when it comes to universal coverage? What role do public hospitals play both in protecting the vulnerable and allowing us to ignore the sources of their vulnerability? Can or should we hope for a day when the public hospital is no longer needed?

A Spirit of Charity has many of the answers to these vital questions.

PREFACE
THE MAJOR PLAYERS

For the purposes of this book, I've focused on the history and current status of five large American public hospitals.

All of them share common traits, but they are also distinctively different, as I hope you'll come to understand. The most common denominator of four of them: They are survivors in a highly competitive health care marketplace where one-third to one-half of their patients have no insurance, or rely on state Medicaid programs to cover their bills. The fifth hospital was orphaned in 2005 after years of neglect.

Let me introduce them:

Grady Memorial Hospital in Atlanta is the primary focus of this narrative because of its long history, the compelling financial and political challenges it continuously faces, and—last but not least—because as an Atlanta journalist, I am most familiar with it. In 2013, Grady listed $93.1 million in charity care in the report it is required to file with the Centers for Medicare & Medicaid Services. While it is the smallest of these hospitals, Grady, which opened in 1892, provides a great prism for the issues I want to illuminate in this book.

Parkland Memorial Hospital in Dallas is similar to Grady and has most recently come out from under intense federal supervision for quality-of-care issues. The new Parkland Hospital that opened in August 2015 is perhaps the most state-of-the-art public hospital in the country. It is testimony as well to the public's willingness to secure its future. In 2013 Parkland reported $316.9 million in charity care in federal filings.

Jackson Memorial Hospital in Miami has faced financial issues similar to Grady's and struggles to maintain its charity mission in a state, like Georgia, that has steadfastly refused to expand health insurance coverage for the poor. Jackson Memorial provided $111.1 million in charity care in 2013.

The John H. Stroger Hospital of Cook County, in Chicago, also known simply as "County" in recognition of the aging facility it replaced in 2002, is among the leaders in experimenting with new methods of health care delivery and payment. The county hospital system, in conjunction with federally funded primary care clinics in and around Chicago and the Illinois Medicaid program, operates an HMO-type insurance plan for low-income residents. County reported charity care costs of $163.3 million in 2013.

And last, **Charity Hospital** of New Orleans, which was closed after Hurricane Katrina in 2005. Founded by Roman Catholic nuns in 1736 and eventually owned by the city and state of Louisiana, Charity was the very definition of an urban hospital dedicated to serving the poor. Charity's doors were padlocked after the storm, even though it could have reopened within weeks. Louisiana officials instead spent the next ten years using disaster relief money to build a new hospital, University Medical Center (UMC), in a once-residential neighborhood nearby. What happens at UMC in the next few years, whether and how its mission of caring for the poor might differ from Charity's, will say a lot about the future of public hospitals and government support for them.

While concentrating on these five, it's important to understand that there are a few dozen other public hospitals like these around the country, hospitals that were chartered by state or local governments to provide vital services to residents without regard for their ability to pay. They include places like New York City's iconic Bellevue Hospital (one month older than Charity), the University of Louisville Hospital, Regional

One Health in Memphis, MetroHealth Medical Center in Cleveland, and the Denver Health Medical Center.

To varying degrees, all of the hospitals in this category rely on public support, usually in the form of tax dollars over and above what they get from Medicare, Medicaid, and private insurance plans. These hospitals, and others like them, show up in this book too.

And then there are hundreds more hospitals that, while not necessarily publicly chartered or financed with tax dollars, continue to provide a significant amount of free and reduced-cost care in the communities they serve. This is especially true of many of the academic medical centers that operate both specialty and community hospitals where doctors get their training.

In early 2015, after the first full year of the Affordable Care Act, about 32 million Americans remained uninsured. Millions of others, while covered for the first time thanks to the 2010 law, hold policies that require them to pay substantial out-of-pocket premiums and expenses that they can ill afford. If they need hospitalization, these hospitals remain their safety net. These people, and the hospitals that serve them, are why this book was written.

INTRODUCTION

"Get your things together. You need to get to Richard quickly."

If the calm tone in her neighbor's voice hadn't shown the urgency of the news, her ashen face left no doubt when Isobel Moutrey opened the front door to her West Atlanta home.

Two other neighbors waited in their car as she gathered her phone, purse, and other essentials before bolting out the door. While they moved swiftly through Atlanta traffic, they told her all they knew: A car plowed into Isobel's husband, Richard, as he and another neighbor were bicycling through Buckhead, an upscale business and residential district. His fellow rider reported by phone that Richard was conscious, but very badly hurt.

Along the way, Isobel got the call that Richard was being transported to Grady Memorial Hospital, located miles to the south in downtown Atlanta.

"Grady? Why not Piedmont?" she thought to herself. Richard had been to the ER at Piedmont Hospital in Buckhead a few years earlier when he hurt himself while working in the yard. She knew Piedmont. It was great. Richard was treated well there. She knew nothing about Grady.

"I knew it was a big public hospital," she said, but she knew very little else about it. Nor did it help her perception of the place when she got to the emergency department and had to go through a metal detector. She was furious, but complied. Then she waited for nearly an hour for word about her husband's condition.

"What kind of place is this?" she recalled asking herself.

Henry W. Grady Memorial Hospital is a fixture in Atlanta, one of the oldest hospitals in the city and the largest public hospital in the state of Georgia. The Grady trauma center, where Richard Beckel was taken, is one of the best, and busiest, in the country.

But, like Isobel Moutrey, most Atlantans know it primarily as the poor people's hospital and for good reason. Two-thirds of Grady's patients don't have enough money to pay their bills, or they rely on Medicaid, the government health insurance plan for the poor. Many of them enter the hospital through the always-crowded emergency department, metal detectors and all. More than 75 percent of Grady's patients are black.

So it was on that Super Bowl Sunday, 2012, that Richard Beckel, a business executive with excellent health insurance, and his Canadian-born wife, Isobel Moutrey, entered somewhat unwillingly into the mysterious world of America's public hospitals. Richard had multiple surgeries. He spent weeks on a ventilator that assisted him with breathing, allowing him slowly to recover from his myriad internal injuries.

Isobel lived through the full Grady experience as well.

When she wasn't at Richard's bedside, she spent most of her time on the surgical recovery floor in one of the hospital's renovated wings. A passkey is required to get into the waiting room there, a security measure she grew to appreciate.

She has nothing but praise for the hospital's medical staff, and she grew close to the families of several patients while Richard was there.

But she also remembers the smell of marijuana in the ER waiting room with its gas-station–like restrooms that smelled of urine and vomit. There were other parts of the hospital that sometimes felt unsafe, she said. She attributed this to an aging facility and Grady's "mission to be open to the poor and vulnerable. It was winter, and the warm building was a haven for the homeless. The staff did their best to patrol any situation that arose," she said.

At his discharge months later, the couple had a much better understanding of how essential Grady was in saving Richard's life. They also learned how important Grady is to metro Atlanta. They now count themselves among the hospital's most vocal advocates.

Truth be told, many Americans don't know much about the large, government-owned and -operated urban hospitals that serve as the provider of last resort to this nation's poor and uninsured. These hospitals emerged within our great cities decades ago with specific missions to care for the "indigent sick," but their importance today seems little understood in the context of the massive changes taking place in our nation's health care system.

We recognize many of them from their iconic names and the regular news coverage that attends them: Bellevue in New York, (Cook) County in Chicago, Jackson Memorial in Miami, and Parkland in Dallas, to name just a few.

Because of Hurricane Katrina, many of us came to know one of the nation's oldest, Charity Hospital in New Orleans. Remarkably, Charity recovered quickly from the storm and flooding, but was unceremoniously abandoned by state and local governments in the aftermath. I shall have much more to say about that in a later chapter.

There are dozens of hospitals like Grady around the country, civic fixtures that once were the largest and most important medical institutions in the community, but places now that those of us with good health insurance would rather avoid.

Yet these are often the same places where thousands of young physicians and nurses were assigned their first on-the-job training. Generations of medical professionals spent long nights and sleepy days in the crowded wards and treatment rooms of these hospitals, suturing wounds, delivering newborns, and—facing the hard truth of medicine—recognizing that they can't save everyone.

It is here that they learned the abbreviated life stories and met the victims of heart attack, stroke, and violent accidents whom they were required to pronounce dead. Yet it was also here—at these places—where they came to understand that the vocation they chose could literally save lives. There is no better place to train than at a public hospital, as many physicians will tell you.

How these hospitals survive, who pays for them, and how they fit into the nation's $3 trillion-a-year health care system is a mystery to most of us.

This is a book about these special places. My goal here is to help interpret their history and significance for general readers and, along the way, to explain why they have come to be the symbol of how the poor are cared for in the United States.

Not surprisingly, in a country that has yet to determine whether access to basic medical care is a right or an earned privilege, these places bear the burden of that indecision. Indeed, their very existence, as we shall see, makes it easy to avoid the discussion altogether.

That's because most of the people who show up in the emergency rooms and clinics of America's public hospitals represent the gaping holes, the ill-conceived compromises, and the unintended consequences resulting from decades of attempts to reform health care in the United States. Even now. Even after the passage and implementation of the Patient Protection and Affordable Care Act, the latest contentious effort to make health care more affordable and accessible.

Deciding Who Should Get Care

To understand the history of public hospitals in America is, in many ways, to understand the contradictions embedded within the American experiment of self-governance. For these places of healing stand in perpetual tension between the highest charitable aspirations of our nation as a whole, and a strong opposing attempt, with roots in state government, to separate the "truly disadvantaged" who deserve help from those who won't take care of themselves.

Nowhere is this more obvious than in the South.

Here it is often difficult to distinguish legitimate disagreement about the cost and effectiveness of government-provided social services from the region's ugly history of government-promoted discrimination. Just consider the political geography on display in a 2015 map of those states that have embraced health care reform and those states that continue to actively oppose it. You can almost see the invisible ink of the defeated Confederate States of America in 1865. It mirrors, as well, the region where the harshest state's-rights battles were waged over desegregation in 1965.

And there's this: The map of the modern South provides an X-ray image of where the population is much more likely to include residents suffering from chronic diseases compared to other regions of the country. These are conditions such as hypertension, diabetes, obesity, and, most recently, new cases of HIV/AIDs, which are endemic among the poor and socially marginalized, both African-American and white. Is this a mere coincidence?

Even without the specter of racism and other enduring forms of discrimination founded in social class, gender, and ethnicity, public hospitals have always existed in the uneasy gap between altruism and austerity when it comes to the appropriation of tax dollars. From a strictly political perspective, these hospitals have been a rich source of patronage jobs for big-city power brokers. Many of them have provided ample reason for public skepticism about their stewardship.

But they have also served as a training camp for generations of public health advocates who demand more attention be paid to the needs of the poor. These voices are important because, while politicians like to talk about "American exceptionalism," they rarely mention how exceptionally different our health care spending priorities are from Europe and other advanced nations.

No doubt America's exceptionalism has spawned great scientific advancements in the detection and treatment of disease. But the reality is that these medical achievements are not shared equally by our citizens. In comparison to other developed nations in preventing disease, disability, and death, we fare poorly while outspending all of them.

What keeps us from doing better, and where do public hospitals fit into this picture?

In medicine, there is a condition among infants called "failure to thrive." Premature birth, infections, and an inability to absorb nutrients are common causes for why some infants do not grow as well as they should. But inconsistent feeding and poverty can cause the condition too. Another important risk factor: The lack of an emotional bond between parent and child.

In many ways, this is what has happened to America's public hospitals and the people they serve. They cannot thrive by relying on the marketplace alone. They need consistent government support. Without it, they are left to bear more and more financial responsibility for caring for an impoverished clientele.

The historic bond between these hospitals and the governments that gave them birth is being challenged in an era of fiscal austerity and reliance on marketplace solutions to health care spending. That is especially so in those states whose hostility to the federal government has caused them to forgo billions of dollars in funding offered under the Affordable Care Act that could have provided coverage for millions of newly insured poor.

Wherever they are located, our great public hospitals represent more than a frayed safety net. They have become also a safety valve for the nation's medical-industrial complex. They exist, not just to take care of the poor, but to relieve others from the challenge to profits that poor people represent. If this country has, as we often hear, "the greatest health care system in the world," it is because these hospitals allow that system to thrive even if they themselves are too often denied the same opportunity.

Here's another way of looking at it: Hospitals that run out of room in their emergency departments go on "diversion," the code word they use to notify ambulance crews to take incoming patients somewhere else. Diversion is an accepted practice in emergency medicine.

But this is also an accepted practice in everyday American medicine. It isn't that privately owned hospitals—whether for-profit or not-for-profit—routinely shut their emergency room doors to poor patients. (Under federal law, they can't turn away a patient with a life-threatening condition. But, once stabilized, they can lawfully send them home.)

Many private hospitals provide a responsible level of financial assistance to those who can't afford it. Still, there is a limit to what they are willing to do, and because of keen competition in the market, they often are on diversion when it comes to taking care of the poor and uninsured when those patients need nonemergency care. In this way, public hospitals have become the pressure release valve for our system.

If they did not exist, we would be forced to invent them. Because they exist—indeed, many, like Grady, have been around for more than a century—we seem content to take them for granted.

Maybe that is understandable. There's often a sense of déjà vu to discussions about how the country's urban charity hospitals are on the brink.

Grady's history in Atlanta, for instance, includes equal parts dysfunctional local governance and a state political leadership that has been studiously indifferent.

Nor are public hospitals always the most accommodating of places. Despite efforts to improve the "consumer experience" by making their facilities more like the competition, a visit to many of them, even the great ones, can feel like a trip to the DMV. Isobel Moutrey's experience with Grady's ER waiting room is all too common.

A Bigger Picture

But a larger, more complete narrative for Grady and so many other hospitals like it must also include numerous examples of excellence in "battlefield" medicine, scientific advancement in clinical care, and the remarkable healing services practiced by generations of physicians, nurses, and staff, all of whom understand their primary mission is to take care of the poor.

Still, this fact remains: Unless you're badly injured, like Richard Beckel, or you're poor, you don't choose to go to Grady.

It wasn't always that way. Not long ago, more babies were born at Grady than at any other hospital in Atlanta. A lot of elderly Atlantans quickly tell you they are "Grady babies." But when pressed, many of them acknowledge that they have not been back there since their mothers took them out of the formerly segregated hospital's all-white, or all-black, maternity wards. They have a choice about where to get their health care now, and for most Atlantans, Grady isn't anywhere near the top of the list.

Just as city fathers predicted in 1892, when the first hospital bearing crusading journalist Henry W. Grady's name opened, Grady is a magnet for the poor, the homeless, and the dispossessed. That's probably fitting for a hospital that was created when the post–Civil War almshouses and infirmaries in Atlanta could not handle the increasing public health load for a growing city.

Even today, from the windows of Grady's long corridors, dozens of homeless men can be seen huddled in blankets on winter nights and seeking shade from the harsh sun on summer afternoons on the streets beneath the shelter of overpasses along the I-75/85 "downtown connector" that bisects Atlanta. It is as if they want to stay close to the one place they know will take them in.

Large numbers of people who have no way of paying for their care visit Grady's outpatient clinics every day to get their high blood pressure or blood sugar levels back under control. The emergency department takes all comers suffering from virtually every disorder of the body and the mind—even if patients know they'll have to wait hours to be seen. Still, they come. Upwards of 435,000 outpatient visits each year (the equivalent of every man, woman, and child who lives in the city of Atlanta), more than 100,000 of them entering through the emergency room.

And it's not just basic medical care they seek, or need. If you are poor, without insurance, and faced with a late diagnosis of advanced cancer, Grady's staff will pull out all stops to get you chemotherapy that might help beat the odds of an early death—the same costly treatment readily available to insured patients in other Atlanta hospitals just a few blocks away. It offers the best stroke care and intervention in the city, even though few people know it.

Most of the Atlanta metro area's five million residents recognize that charity is at the heart of Grady's mission and that it gets some local funding from county governments. They know, too, that it is the go-to trauma hospital for the region, which is why Richard Beckel was taken there. Local newscasts routinely set up cameras outside the Grady ER to chronicle the mayhem on Atlanta's streets and carnage from its highways.

Television commercials, roadside billboards, and placards on grocery carts tout the lifesaving work of Grady's trauma doctors and nurses. Richard Beckel's picture is on some of those placards.

But metro Atlanta residents are largely unaware of Grady's critical role in training many of the doctors who work in the hospitals where the more affluent gravitate; or how Grady's comprehensive HIV/AIDS clinic is a model for others around the country; or that Grady has the only sickle-cell clinic in the region; or that it houses the state's most advanced unit for people who suffer life-threatening burns. They understand even less about how the hospital and its services are financed, and how it can afford to provide all that free care. What they do hear, all too frequently, is how it is on the brink of insolvency or in political turmoil over how it is managed.

The social and policy issues Grady raises are complex and cut across all levels of government. They are infused with local politics—rural versus urban, or frugal Republican suburbs versus tax-and-spend city Democrats.

And then there's the issue of race, always race, especially with Grady's history of separate and not-always-equal treatment of the city's large African-American population. These and other issues invariably surface when talk turns to Grady.

If you see similarities to this debate where you live, it is probably because there is a Grady that operates on a similar knife-edge of viability in your city.

Even after full implementation of the 2010 Patient Protection and Affordable Care Act—the latest effort at reform—public hospitals still remain the only hope for millions of Americans left without health insurance coverage. And, like Grady, they may be running out of ways to adapt.

Insurance companies, pharmaceutical firms, and other segments of the medical-industrial complex have proven quite successful at navigating the changing currents of health policy over the decades. They will find ways to prosper with this most recent reform effort as well. But history shows public hospitals are always among the last to benefit from the very changes supposedly designed to make the overall system more affordable and equitable. Time and again, reform after reform, they find themselves waiting to see how the larger market responds, and then creating new ways to care for—and pay for—the patients still left behind.

And there are always patients left behind.

Nearly a century ago, after Germany, England, and other European countries enacted compulsory health insurance, the United States rejected the idea, despite evidence that the rising cost of medical care was jeopardizing the welfare of working-class families. Powerful forces—corporations, unions, physicians, and insurance companies—helped torpedo the concept, arguing that voluntary plans would suffice. Although some of the players have changed positions, and new ones have joined the fray, there has been no serious effort since then to make health insurance universally available to every American.

Reform efforts instead have been aimed at making health care more affordable and available to one group at a time, as sociologist Paul Starr has noted. Periodic reform efforts have also been designed to pacify employers, insurance companies, doctors, hospitals, and other major players, all the while hiding the true cost of care to many Americans, Starr says.

These incremental steps have also generated intense debate and, at times, resulted in policies that have unintended consequences.

For instance, in the New Deal era, the movement toward voluntary group health insurance was started exclusively to help pay hospital bills, not doctor bills. The impact of that initial determination—that health insurance is primarily a hedge against the high cost of hospital care—would haunt the health care system for decades to come, not because it wasn't true at the time, but because in later years, it became much harder to switch gears and underwrite coverage for primary care and preventive services to help keep people *out* of the hospital.

How We Got Here

Another round of reforms enacted fifty years ago with the creation of Medicare set the stage for where we are now.

Medicare was established to guarantee care to the nation's oldest and most vulnerable patients. And it has unquestionably worked, improving access to health care, extending lives, and, along with Social Security, assuring the elderly and disabled that they will not have to choose between paying medical bills and putting food on the table—a harsh reality for millions of Americans prior to 1965. (It's also worth noting that the United States is the only country in the world to create a compulsory health insurance plan that benefits only the elderly. Virtually every other developed nation has universal coverage for all its citizens.)

Even by singling out only one segment of its population, the sweeping federal program still fundamentally altered how health care is delivered and who provides it in our country.

Backed by federal payroll taxes, Medicare provided the financial footing for a burgeoning market of for-profit and non-profit hospitals, many of them built with the help of federal construction money in the decades before the law was passed. And, most importantly, because it paid for care in a growing population of Americans who up until then couldn't afford it, Medicare allowed most of the health care system to narrow its vision of how much charity care was needed for the poor and uninsured.

A marketplace adjustment such as Medicare could have been absorbed, probably without long-term problems, except that the country failed to fully take the next step—to set up a similar program for the poor.

Here is where most Americans can be forgiven for being confused. Isn't Medicaid the program for the poor? Isn't it run by the same federal agency that runs Medicare?

Answering this is essential to understanding the policy issues coming to bear on America's public hospitals. (I'll be elaborating on them in subsequent chapters.)

Put simply, it is critical to understand that, unlike Medicare, Medicaid never received a designated source of revenue to make it sustainable as a legitimate health care program for the poor. In order to get enough votes to levy payroll taxes that would allow the federal government to run the health care program for the elderly, President Lyndon B. Johnson and Medicare's promoters gave the fifty states much more leeway in the creation of Medicaid and how it is financed. This tactic showed the kind of political savvy that made Johnson so successful in the legislative arena. Medicare, after all, was the prize. It was the leftover piece of the progressive agenda that went back to the Franklin D. Roosevelt era and the genesis of Social Security.

But the deal-making over Medicare by LBJ and his legislative adjutants also pinpoints the spot where Medicaid's trajectory veered off mission, and why every new reform effort since then has also run off the rails when it attempted to deal with health care for the poor.

This 1965 compromise between the federal government and the states spawned drastic disparities in how much states spend on Medicaid, whom they choose to cover, and what kinds of health services they provide. (For Medicare, the federal government makes those decisions.) Indeed, it was left up to the states to decide whether they even wanted to be included in the program, and many of them initially balked. (Arizona was the last state to get on board, but that was seventeen years after the law was passed.)

While participation in Medicaid requires states to provide a baseline of mandatory coverage to some special categories of the poor, it does not extend coverage to individuals in low-paying jobs, or part-time workers, or those who are temporarily out of work, the way unemployment benefits can be used by workers who are laid off.

Congress has approved some changes to those baseline eligibility rules over the years. Low-income pregnant women can get coverage, along with their children. Elderly and disabled Americans who qualify for Medicare can get nursing home and doctor coverage under Medicaid if they exhaust their cash resources. But for the most part, Medicaid is off-limits to able-bodied Americans, whether they are working or not.

Despite being so stingy with eligibility, benefits, and reimbursements, state spending on Medicaid has steadily grown over the years, the result of swings in the economy, long-term unemployment trends, and the same escalating costs of medical services that plague Medicare and private insurance plans. The result is that Medicaid is one of the biggest items in state budgets. For some governors and legislators, it is their favorite whipping post. They argue it crowds out spending for schools, prisons, highways, and other programs that have more widespread political support. So they try to spend as little on it as possible, or find ways to get the federal government to pick up more of the tab.

Because states get to set the reimbursement rate for doctors and hospitals taking care of Medicaid patients—and because often those rates don't even cover the cost of treatment, let alone overhead—many physicians simply refuse to accept Medicaid patients. That refusal, which is the direct result of state budget-makers' shortchanging the program over the years, allows Medicaid's opponents to condemn it as unworkable and ineffective. As a political tactic, starving a social program like Medicaid, unemployment insurance, and food stamps, and then claiming they don't work, has a rich history in the Southern states.

For most American hospitals, low reimbursement is more of an annoyance than a threat. Medicaid is a relatively insignificant source of revenue, dwarfed certainly in comparison with Medicare, but also by hundreds of private insurers paying the bills of the vast majority of their patients. Still, it's easy to see why nonprofit hospitals get antsy about treating too many Medicaid patients.

Even so, it is Medicaid that represents the single largest source of revenue for many public hospitals like Grady. And when combined with those patients who have no means of paying whatsoever—no government or private insurance and no bank account to draw on—Medicaid and charity care often account for more than half of public hospitals' patients.

As accountants might say, that's a toxic business model. Indeed, this defining characteristic of treating such a high volume of uninsured and Medicaid patients is what sets apart these large, urban hospitals from thousands of other institutions around the country that are routinely called "safety-net" hospitals.

Many nonprofit and government-owned hospitals claim safety-net status, most of them because they may be the only providers of comprehensive health services in their community. But the volume of paying patients they treat usually more than offsets the cost of providing charity care. There are far fewer—less than 100 of the approximately 4,000 hospitals nationwide—that treat high numbers of Medicaid patients. And there are only a handful of these, like Grady, where the majority of their patients have no insurance or are covered by Medicaid.

The only way the public hospitals in this last group can make up for such a poor mix of patients is to turn, time and again, to the local or state governments that subsidize their operations. And local elected officials—not unlike their counterparts at the federal level—are not looking for reasons to raise taxes, especially in an economy that, in many areas, has yet to rebound to what real property values were prior to the 2008 recession.

Local elected officials can be forgiven for suggesting this is mostly Washington's problem.

But in the halting attempts to reform the nation's health care system in the years since Medicare and Medicaid were established, improving access to insurance for the poor has never really been front and center.

There have been a few attempts to expand Medicare to cover anyone who can't afford private insurance and, unlike the elderly, charge a sliding scale premium based on income, the way low-income people can qualify for housing vouchers. But those ideas have been tossed aside as unworkable, or too expensive at best, and a step toward European-style socialized health care at worst. (It isn't anything of the sort, but even advocates of national health insurance have been quick to say the country isn't quite ready for this yet.)

Affordability over Expanding Coverage

Instead, policy efforts have concentrated on the affordability, fairness, and efficiency of the commercial insurance market for employers who cover their workers with group plans and individuals who buy on the private market. Politically speaking, it has always been easier to get voters agitated about health care reform when the premiums for their group health plans keep going up, their out-of-pocket expenses continue to rise, and their benefits get reduced.

Yet even those meager efforts have met stubborn resistance from the health care industry, whose greatest triumph was the sacking of President Bill Clinton and First Lady Hillary Clinton's reform efforts in his first term. The Clintons did succeed at opening up public financing to expand access for children's health insurance late in his second term, but not without granting considerable leeway to the states to determine what level of family income qualified for the subsidized plans.

So many health care advocates watched with considerable anticipation as President Barack Obama broke through the decades-old antipathy toward Medicaid and included a major expansion of the program to cover the working poor as part of the Affordable Care Act in 2010. For the first time, Americans earning above the poverty level—but still not enough to buy a private insurance policy, even with a subsidy—would qualify for Medicaid.

Underwriters calculated that as many as half of the estimated fifty million Americans who were without insurance in 2010 when the law was passed could be covered by the greatly expanded Medicaid program. Most of the rest should be able to buy subsidized insurance plans on a private market that, also for the first time, could no longer exclude high-risk people from coverage or deny them care once they got sick.

The linchpin for that last reform—the one that forbade insurance companies from excluding applicants they thought might cost them too much—was the requirement that every individual must purchase a health plan or face a fine when it came time to settle up on their federal taxes. Opponents of the 2010 law, including virtually every Republican in Congress, saw the individual mandate as their best chance to mount a constitutional challenge to the new reform effort. Their opposition to requiring states to expand Medicaid was almost an afterthought. And, within months, the law landed on the Supreme Court's docket.

It's easy to forget now that in 2012 the high court found relatively easy agreement with the states on the Medicaid challenge to the Affordable Care Act. However, it upheld the overall law, including the individual mandate, as constitutional by a contentious 5–4 vote.

Ruling separately in the same case, seven of the nine justices declared the federal government had overreached in demanding the states provide millions of Americans new and easier access to Medicaid. The court declared the ACA was "coercive" in that it was essentially forcing the states to give up their traditional role in determining who qualified for Medicaid coverage. States should determine for themselves whether they want to opt into expanding Medicaid, the court said; Congress could not force them to do so.

As legal scholars have since noted, the ruling was in keeping with a string of high-court decisions over the years calling into question the uneasy relationship between the state and federal governments around Medicaid, with the states gaining increasing legal leverage at almost every turn. But the 2012 ruling reinforced, this time with enormous impact, Medicaid's bastard-child role in the still-unfinished business of providing universal access to health insurance for all Americans.

The cost of this one decision—not to mention all the other legislative, regulatory, and policy shortcomings in reform efforts over the years—can be measured in real dollars, disability, and death. Lack of insurance cost 18,000 American lives in the year

2000, according to the Institute of Medicine. A more recent estimate prior to the adoption of the ACA put the body count as high as 45,000 yearly, according to researchers at Harvard Medical School and the Cambridge Health Alliance. This happens in a country that prides itself for having the best medical care in the world. There is no other industrialized nation where such a staggering annual death toll is linked to lack of access due to lack of insurance.

Caught in the Trap

Which brings us back to Grady.

After barely escaping insolvency in 2008 with a change in governance and new leadership, Grady's leaders had hoped the 2010 health reform law would usher in a period of financial stability and continued improvements to the massive facility in the heart of downtown Atlanta.

Political appointees who long made it a patronage mill for friends and cronies were no longer running the place, having finally yielded control to a nonprofit corporation of local business and civic leaders. Grady started getting millions of dollars from foundations, individuals, and other philanthropies for long-deferred capital improvements. The community had high hopes that with the passage of the ACA the mix of patients and payers would finally get to the point where the hospital could support itself and plan for the future.

Instead, several independent trends have coincided to place a large question mark over Grady's future—and that of other hospitals like it around the country. About the same time Grady began its reformation, a huge upsurge of mentally ill patients descended on it. These were seriously ill patients dispossessed by federal court order because state mental hospitals were understaffed, underfunded, and jeopardizing their lives.

Virtually every public hospital in the United States has experienced this surge of behavioral health patients who show up in their ERs, often without insurance, in need of hospitalization.

Because of new payment mechanisms that made treating certain types of trauma cases more lucrative, there is some fear that other hospitals in the Atlanta metro region will begin to siphon off patients gravely injured on the job or on the highways, patients that were once Grady's alone. This could leave Grady to handle what some urban hospitals call the knife-and-gun club, the shootings and stabbings, featuring patients unlikely to bring an insurance card with them into trauma center triage. Florida is already seeing this trend as for-profit hospitals in the suburbs of its major cities have been allowed to set up trauma services.

And, since illegal immigrants are specifically forbidden from coverage under the ACA, no one else routinely treats metro Atlanta's substantial undocumented population. That's still left to Grady as well as its large urban counterparts around the country, according to America's Essential Hospitals, an organization that represents safety-net hospitals around the country.

Yet it is the political issue of Medicaid—and the state's decision to refuse an estimated $9 million a day in federal funds to expand it—that has raised the prospect of leaving Grady behind once again. Within days of the Supreme Court's ruling in 2012, Georgia's political leaders said they were walking through the exit door provided by the court's ruling and opting out of Medicaid expansion. Opposition to the ACA and Medicaid in almost any form, not just to the expansion, has since become an organizing principle for the state's Republican leadership.

Nineteen states (most of them in the South) continue to show little interest in expanding Medicaid to the working poor, as the ACA envisioned.

This is more than another chapter in the South's well-documented antipathy to ensuring that poor people have adequate access to health care. Indeed, in the nation as a whole, public

opinion over the role played by the federal government in securing health care coverage for all citizens flip-flopped between
2006 and 2014, and not in the way one might have expected.

Prior to President Obama's election in 2008, a bellwether
Gallup survey found that, by a margin of more than two to one
(69 percent to 29 percent), Americans believed the federal government should guarantee coverage for all. But by the end of
2014, just as the new law that strives to do that was being fully
implemented, fewer than half of Americans surveyed (42 percent) felt the federal government has this responsibility, while
the majority of those surveyed (52 percent) said there should
be no such guarantee. The reversal speaks volumes about how
toxic the topic can become and why politicians would rather
avoid it.

Yet, as the result of this continuing uncertainty, Georgia is
once again putting at risk Grady's long-standing role as a teaching hospital for one in four doctors practicing in Georgia. It is
limiting Grady's ability to operate the largest trauma care center in the Southeast and provide the best and most advanced
treatment of HIV/AIDs, stroke care, neonatal intensive care,
and other much-needed community services. I'll spend some
time examining those services and how they are paid for in
this book.

For a hospital that was long known as "the Gradys"—
meaning that it maintained separate hospitals for whites and
blacks for years, and separate-but-unequal wings for blacks and
whites when the most recent hospital opened in 1958—dealing
with the latest ideological skirmish over how to care for the
poor may prove to be its most difficult challenge ever.

Public hospitals in Dallas, Miami, Tampa, Nashville,
Birmingham, New Orleans, Memphis, Charleston, and other
cities, mostly in the South—all operating in states that have
decided not to expand Medicaid—face similar challenges to
provide costly, essential services not available to the poor at
competing hospitals. Public health advocates in these cities

understand that if the reverse were true—if the public hospitals were to be closed, and their poor and uninsured patients diverted to other hospitals—a sea of red ink could overwhelm even those private hospitals that are now more prosperous.

In the last decade alone, D.C. General in Washington, Charity in New Orleans, and Martin Luther King Jr./Charles Drew in Los Angeles—all similar to Grady, all serving mostly minority communities—have shuttered their doors, forcing new ways of treating the poor and uninsured at other institutions with varying degrees of success. They closed for a host of reasons, including lack of state and local funding, uncertainty in Washington, and rank mismanagement from local governments and hospital administrations that were supposed to ensure their survival.

Others have haltingly adapted to the ever-changing health care marketplace, becoming huge "systems," with multiple hospitals and outpatient clinics, merging with county health departments, and even, in a handful of cities, becoming insurers by establishing health maintenance organizations for their Medicaid clients. The results of these efforts are harder to measure—other than to note that the hospitals have, at least, survived through the turmoil of our latest policy changes. A few are showing signs of revitalization.

Still, there is great concern that the headlong rush toward restructuring public hospitals in ways that make them look and act like their nonprofit and private competitors will inevitably challenge their original mission of serving the poor.

But know this too: America's public hospitals are remarkable at survival. Some of the best and brightest minds in medicine, management, and administration are committed to the cause of caring for the poor.

The hospitals where they work are sentinels for the future of health care in America. Knowing more about them will improve the discussion of health care reform as we move forward.

PART I
POOR PEOPLE PLACES

It wasn't so much the periodic outbreaks of yellow fever, or the neighborhoods plagued by dysentery from tainted water supplies, or even the disabled veterans of the Civil War that created the need for the first publicly financed hospitals in America's big cities.

And it wasn't as if other well-intentioned approaches had not been tried. The Roman Catholic nuns who came from Ireland and France to care for America's poor, as well as the good Christian men and women of Protestant churches, struggled mightily to make good their mission of providing meals and a bed in almshouses and giving comfort care to the sick and infectious in what became known as "pesthouses."

It was the cities themselves that created a new magnitude of need. They were teeming with people, yellow fever, and cholera in the midst of poor public health. Charity alone would no longer suffice.

Southern cities, in particular, had become a refuge for freed slaves and their families, looking to start new lives away from the plantations. The sons and daughters of white farmers—not from the plantation elite, but the dirt farmers who could no longer make a living off their family's land—joined them. In other parts of the country, the cities attracted a growing workforce that tended the fires of the nation's industrial revolution where the risk of injury was high.

By the beginning of America's second century in the late nineteenth century, the foundries and carpet mills, factories, and slaughterhouses in major cities—all connected by railroads and rivers that transported goods, people, and diseases like a continent-wide circulatory system—triggered a shift in the nation's population from rural countryside to crowded cities. Few of these urban areas were capable of providing the public health and medical care their new dwellers needed.

Something else was happening as well during this time. Science was slowly taking hold on the practice of medicine.

In the early decades of the nineteenth century, the professional status of doctors ascended. They were moving from being often-passive assistants in the healing powers of nature, to serving as clinical practitioners with advanced training in pathology and anatomy. They examined patients and began to record, in some detail, the therapies they prescribed.

Accompanying that first wave of urbanization came another set of practitioners trained in surgical techniques to remove diseased tissue and reduce the risk of infection. They were even able to do so without the patient being awake and in gruesome pain. Equally important, women, trained in the first formal schools of nursing, began to take the place of an earlier age's missionary nuns at the bedside of patients, lessening the need for family members to be pressed into service as caregivers.

All of these skills were employed in makeshift battlefield facilities during the Civil War and in military hospitals, where doctors and surgeons were saving the lives of seriously wounded soldiers who would have been left for dead in previous conflicts.

In the decades immediately after the war, physicians achieved enough status that businessmen and political leaders began to listen to them. For the first time, practitioners raised the subject of the connection between social conditions and the causes of disease.

America began to discover it wanted—and needed—hospitals.

Antibiotics and vaccines had not yet lessened the toll that

bacteria and viruses caused when disease outbreaks could still wipe out whole sections of cities. Human decency and public health demanded a more determined and publicly financed response. In city after city, almshouses became hospitals; pesthouses became infirmaries; and the newly established medical and nursing schools found in them a place for education and training.

Most importantly, with these new medical procedures gaining attention, the wealthy sought out services that could only be performed in an institution, by a physician, accompanied by nurses. For decades, when the business and political elite of the cities were injured or ill, local physicians were called to their homes to make them better. Now they were more likely to go to a hospital where the doctor had access to a growing armamentarium of drugs, devices, and surgical procedures.

Not coincidentally, then, this was also the time when American medicine recorded the first calls to separate the poor from everyone else. Nearly everyone agreed the poor must be cared for. It simply wouldn't do to have them dying in the streets.

But if cities were to provide free health care for the poor, would that not encourage more of the sick and destitute to relocate to the cities and prolong the problem?

Wouldn't such a commitment to charity care place a bigger burden on municipal treasuries that were needed for other necessities such as roads, schools, or even sanitary sewers to keep people from getting sick in the first place?

Should the poor be entitled to the same level of care as those who could responsibly pay on their own?

And if cities found these hospitals necessary, what would their minimum level of funding be?

Over the course of the next 150 years, America would confront those questions many times in public-policy debates at the local, state, and national levels. It has yet to fully answer them.

IS CHARITY CARE A MISSION OR IS IT THE LAW?
A Q&A on Public Hospital Financing

Do all public hospitals have to provide unlimited charity care?
For most large public hospitals in the United States, especially those created by cities and state governments in the nineteenth and early twentieth centuries, there is language in their charters requiring them to provide care to residents who can't afford it. These patients are often referred to in authorizing legislation as the "indigent sick." The city of Atlanta's ordinance "accepting" the still-under-construction Grady Memorial Hospital in 1891 uses this terminology.

In return for treating these patients, the city pledges to "support and maintain" the hospital, although in the Grady ordinance, for example, the city does not stipulate how it will go about doing that. Over the years, Grady's deal with the city included the city providing free water services for the hospital. That arrangement continues even though the city long ago turned the hospital over to a separate hospital authority. Many of the public hospitals must also provide free care to police and firefighters, even in nonemergency situations.

Some of the authorizing legislation creating public hospitals provides more specifics about required specialized services, such as trauma care and burn care, but most don't. These expensive services have evolved at public hospitals over the years, and the general appropriations they get from local governments and states rarely cover the full cost of providing them.

How much of the hospitals' operating budgets are the governments supposed to pick up?

Many of the deals struck between local and state governments and public hospitals are ambiguous when it comes to public funding. But the longer the relationship, the more likely the marriage between charity care and public funding becomes part of the hospital's DNA, even if it is not stipulated in their contracts.

Larry Gage, the former chief executive officer of the National Association of Public Hospitals (now known as America's Essential Hospitals) is an expert on these arrangements between governing authorities and the hospitals they support. The government's pledge almost always includes helping the hospital raise money for capital improvements through tax-exempt bonds. But it often extends to direct funding for operations as well. Sometimes the hospital simply provides a bill to the government entity for the total cost of indigent care and then settles for a portion of that.

More recently, especially as hospitals have reorganized, local officials are demanding the hospitals specifically account not just for how much they expect local taxpayers to put out, but also how the hospital is spending their appropriated funds.

How do the hospitals and their government sponsors balance the mission of providing charity care with prudent spending of taxpayer dollars?

There are many ways to do this. Most public hospitals negotiate a yearly amount with the government that supports them. This usually is based on a "cost-plus" scale (the cost of providing the care, plus a small—up to 2 percent—markup). But often the language in these contracts about the responsibility of the hospital and the payments required by the local governments is vague.

Gage points to the statute creating the Denver Health and Hospital Authority, which includes specific language granting "access to qualified, preventive acute and chronic health care for all citizens of Denver regardless of ability to pay." But the operating contract it has with the city also requires the authority to quantify the cost of the services and how much the city is responsible for paying.

Rather than an open-ended requirement to provide services for all indigent patients, the contract between Harbor View Hospital in Seattle and the county applies to patients in eleven "priority groups." These include jail inmates, the involuntarily committed mentally ill, substance abusers, patients with sexually transmitted diseases, trauma and burn victims, and "non–English-speaking poor."

The hospital gets no direct operational money from the county. Instead, it calls for "priority for care within the resources available," which indicates that if the hospital runs out of money, it could impose restrictions on how much it spends.

How are tax funds raised locally for public hospitals?
The short answer is lots of different ways. Here are some:
- A property tax levy to support the hospital or a public health department or both
- A sales tax, usually less than 1 percent, the proceeds of which go directly to the hospital or is passed through the local government
- A general appropriation from the local government's operating budget
- Special fees or service charges, such as a fee on motor vehicle licenses to support trauma care networks

Bear in mind that many public hospitals in the United States receive no revenue from any of these types of local taxes. Instead, they rely on government-backed bonds to help them with capital projects and, on rare occasions, to use for operating expenses.

Aren't VA hospitals considered public hospitals?

Yes, but they are financed and run by the Department of Veterans Affairs, a federal agency, and get no local funding. Many VA hospitals, like local public hospitals, are teaching hospitals too. But VA hospitals are usually restricted to veterans, active military personnel, and military retirees under the age of sixty-five.

If public hospitals are owned by local governments, are the employees hired by and paid by city and county personnel departments?

Most public hospitals have organized as separate, quasi-government agencies that are allowed to hire, fire, and set salaries. They did this specifically to remove constraints on personnel and procurement procedures. Yet because they have contracts with city, county, and state governments to provide a service, many must abide by local ordinances imposed on contractors.

The contract Grady Hospital has with Fulton County, for instance, requires specific minority contracting practices it must use if the county is to back construction bonds for capital projects.

1

AMERICA'S CITIES
AND THEIR HOSPITALS

Born in Dublin, the daughter of devout Catholics, Esther Carroll seemed destined for two things—to become a nun and to be a teacher. When she was twenty-three, she professed her vows with the Sisters of Mercy, a Catholic religious order committed to parish work and philanthropy to the growing Irish population in port cities in the Southern states. And indeed, after arriving in Savannah in 1858, the new Sister Mary Cecilia spent the next seventeen years teaching, much of it in the immediate aftermath of Union Army General William T. Sherman's famous march of destruction from Atlanta to her beautiful new home city on the Georgia coast.

But in 1875, when Sister Mary Cecelia was forty-two, and with no real formal training in medicine, the Bishop of Savannah changed her mission. She and four other Mercy nuns were assigned to a local infirmary that faced wave after wave of patients stricken during epidemics of tropical diseases and other life-threatening infections.

Savannah Hospital, where the nuns worked, is thought to be the earliest real hospital in Georgia. Founded in 1808, it was a part of the nation's first, publicly financed health care system, the United States Marine Hospital Service. Signed into law by President John Adams ten years earlier, "to provide relief and maintenance of disabled Seamen," about three-dozen hospitals, like the one in Savannah, were created over a period of twenty years at seaports and river ports in growing cities. To pay for them, the country's merchant marines were taxed twenty cents a month that went into the Marine Hospital Fund, in effect creating the first health care and disease prevention agency of the federal government.

The decision to create marine hospitals came about the same time the new country faced the reality that global trade—defined at this stage as shipping lanes between Cuba, the Caribbean, Central America, and South America—carried disease, as well as desirable commercial products, to the nation's growing port cities.

Among the most persistent of these threats was yellow fever, a hemorrhagic disease infecting humans through mosquitoes. Yellow fever was easy to spread and difficult to cure.

The nation had experienced outbreaks before, the worst being in Philadelphia in 1793, then-seat of the new government. President George Washington and much of the population were forced to abandon the city during the summer. The epidemic claimed five thousand lives, or about 10 percent of Philadelphia's population.

Every year there seemed to be at least one outbreak of yellow fever in one or two places around the country.

The disease came back with a vengeance in the 1870s, when commerce resumed in the South after the Civil War. In Memphis, where the pathogen was transferred via steamboat and other traffic up the Mississippi from New Orleans, the city was hit with what local historians still describe as an epidemic in 1878 of "biblical proportions." One estimate was that the disease caused 60 percent of the city's population to flee, and it infected most of the rest who stayed. By the end of 1878, Memphis recorded 5,150 yellow fever deaths in that year alone.

It could have been much worse.

Those who got sick in Memphis went to a public hospital, originally chartered in 1829 by the Tennessee legislature. The state appropriated $3,300 to get the hospital set up to deal with periodic outbreaks of yellow fever, cholera, and other infectious diseases. But by 1866, after the war, the state funds dried up. The city of Memphis purchased the facility and levied a tax that raised $11,000 annually to support it. Had Memphis Hospital not been around at the time of the 1878 epidemic, the city would have suffered even more mortality than it did.

Yet while Memphis had invested in a public hospital, it was not in a position to do much else about public health. At the time of the epidemic, there was no city sewer system, and water was still collected in cisterns. It had a reputation as the unhealthiest city in the country.

At the Savannah hospital, Sister Mary Cecilia and her fellow nuns encountered a similar outbreak of yellow fever. Gravely ill patients flooded the cramped wards of the old marine hospital to the point that attic space was needed to care for them. Not surprisingly, the patients treated in the attic, which was accessible only by a rope ladder, and with no water service, were black.

One account of the outbreak puts the death toll in Savannah at 276 in a forty-eight-hour period in 1876. In order to prevent a panic in the city, the corpses were transported at night through a tunnel burrowed under some of Savannah's finest homes. They exited the underground passage in a heavily wooded area in one of the city's famous squares, where the bodies were dispatched in the dead of night to local cemeteries that had no public accounting of their burial. (There was a theory that, like the plague, yellow fever could be spread by contact with the bodies of those who died from the disease.)

The nuns were quick learners and made impressive progress battling the disease. But, at the same time, they were horrified by conditions at the hospital. On their own, the Sisters of Mercy assembled a makeshift pump that was able to deliver water to the patients in the attic, even if they continued to climb a rope to reach them.

Women with a Mission

Sister Mary Cecilia and her nuns began campaigning within Savannah's large Irish-Catholic community to raise money to rebuild the hospital and improve conditions for all its patients. When they raised enough to essentially rebuild the hospital, they gave thanks and renamed it after St. Joseph.

As the yellow fever epidemic spread (they treated more than 550 patients in the 1876 epidemic alone), the hospital took in everyone who needed help, not just mariners. Four hundred and forty survived—a remarkable feat for a disease that was so hard to control.

In so doing, the Sisters of Mercy in Georgia followed in the footsteps of the Sisters of Charity in Louisiana, who took over one of the nation's oldest hospitals in New Orleans in 1832. One hundred years earlier, the hospital had been founded by a French ship builder, who stipulated his estate should go toward building a hospital specifically for the poor in what was then a French colony.

Together with the city, the nuns managed what was to become one of the nation's best-known public hospitals— Charity Hospital in New Orleans—for more than a century. Their legacy would stand until 2005 as one of the oldest, continuously run public hospitals in the United States. (The oldest, Bellevue Hospital, was opened only months earlier in 1736 in a six-bed ward of the New York City Almshouse.)

The work of the Sisters of Mercy in Savannah didn't go unnoticed by businessmen and religious leaders in Atlanta, which was rebuilding quickly after the war.

In 1880, the Bishop of Savannah moved Sister Mary Cecilia to Atlanta, which was battling its own set of public health demons. With her were three other Sisters of Mercy. Among them, legend has it, they had fifty cents in their possession; but, as they had proven in Savannah, they had fund-raising skills. Within months, they would purchase a two-story house and establish Atlanta's first city hospital, enlisting the services of four physicians to their cause. They renamed the ten-bed infirmary after its counterpart in Savannah, St. Joseph's.

With Atlanta's population nearing forty thousand residents, St. Joseph's was immediately overwhelmed with patients, and, just as in Savannah, almost all of them were white, even though the diseases they fought did not discriminate on the basis of race.

In the decades after the Civil War and Reconstruction, Southern cities like Atlanta struggled to survive and establish their own identities. Business leaders, bankers, and crusading journalists hoping to attract commerce pushed for improvements in public education, roads, and, increasingly, public health.

Their concern—borne out by what was happening in the overcrowded wards of almshouses, sanatoriums, and infirmaries—was that charity care would not be enough. Eventually, local government would need to get involved in the form of building, or at least subsidizing, a hospital to deal with the routine scourges of yellow fever, malaria, and dysentery.

Memphis Hospital, Charity in New Orleans, Louisville City Hospital—all of them funded with the help of city or state taxes (and the continued presence of the Sisters of Charity, Sisters of Mercy, and other religious women)—set the pace. But, as sociologist and medical historian Paul Starr has pointed out, these public efforts were not always the result of progressive thinking. Some were created to separate the sick from the poor and dependent. City and state leaders seemed happy to provide a safe haven for the "respectable" poor. But these facilities also were open to affluent city residents who came down with illnesses with a chance for cure.

Atlanta, which was to become poster child of the emerging "New South," had yet to tackle the issue when Sister Mary Cecilia arrived on her new medical mission from Savannah.

That was about to change.

Preaching from a Print Pulpit

Henry Woodfin Grady, born in Athens, Georgia, and educated at the University of Georgia, made a name for himself as a crusading journalist and progressive thinker after the war. In 1880, Grady borrowed $20,000 to buy a partial ownership of one of the city's daily newspapers, *The Constitution*, and became the managing editor. What the Sisters of Mercy practiced in the wards of St. Joseph's, Henry Grady was prepared to preach in the words of his pulpit in *The Constitution*.

In the 1880s, *The Constitution* had a national weekly edition with nearly 150,000 subscribers. Grady's editorials were reprinted there and in smaller newspapers around the country. His journalistic sermons were about commerce and the need for Atlanta to build a "brave and beautiful" new city, putting the war behind it, creating opportunity for freed blacks and girding itself to compete against the North in industry and the movement of agricultural products.

His exhortations clearly had an impact. Northern investors showed up with money. Atlanta began to grow. It hosted the International Cotton Exposition in 1881 and Piedmont Expositions in 1887 and 1889. These were large, international gatherings attracting tens of thousands of visitors to showcase Atlanta, which was quickly becoming the envy of the South. Surely, a city that rebuilt itself so successfully from the ashes of Sherman's fires and led the way for the economic transformation of the South could also find a way to protect its citizens from disease and disability, Grady asked on more than one occasion.

Grady wasn't a lone voice in calling for a government role in health care for those who need it. Others took up the cause with even more vigor. The Atlanta Benevolent Home, one of the first almshouses in the city, persuaded city leaders in 1886 to pay it sixteen cents per day, per resident, to provide medical help for the sick and needy. It wasn't much, but it established a precedent.

A few years after St. Joseph's opened, a group of women teamed up with the new Southern Medical College to open the Ivy Street Hospital. The new facility pioneered emergency medicine in the city. But its most remarkable accomplishment is that it admitted all comers, regardless of ability to pay, including blacks. Eventually when the women who founded it transferred operations to the medical college, the physicians secured an understanding that they could use the hospital for their private patients. In return, the ladies said, the physicians must treat indigent patients at no cost.

The doctors took the deal, but quickly turned to the city for help. They wouldn't be able to keep the hospital open, the doctors said, without a subsidy to pay for all of the indigents who had begun to show up at their doors.

Having already agreed to help care for the sick at the Benevolent Home, the city could see a worrisome trend developing. It surveyed St. Joseph's and other hospitals and infirmaries operating in Atlanta and determined that all of them relied almost exclusively on philanthropic backing to stay open. It agreed to Ivy Street's petition, but came to the conclusion that the other hospitals would eventually expect the same treatment.

It's impossible to determine from historical records how much of a subsidy the city provided Ivy Street. There is only evidence to show that whatever it amounted to, it was much less than what the medical school doctors were getting from their private patients. But it is interesting to note that in 1886 Atlanta, as well as in other cities around the country by this time, the notion that a hospital agreeing to serve the poor would need a government subsidy to survive had already taken firm root. That assumption remains true to this day.

Yet Ivy Street, even with the city subsidy, was not a charity hospital in the classic use of that word to describe public hospitals, or even the old Marine Hospital Service. Even with the city subsidy, Ivy Street relied on income from private-pay patients to offset the cost of services it offered to the poor. Nor were the doors of the other hospitals in Atlanta closed off to poor patients, or even blacks—although all of them, if they took in black patients, housed them separately from whites.

And, as the city expected, all of the hospitals eventually came asking for help. Unfortunately for the hospitals, the city made promises that it could not keep, and, over time, the small subsidies they got grew smaller and could no longer be guaranteed.

It was about this time that Grady and other businessmen in Atlanta started calling for a new approach—a city hospital like those in Memphis, New Orleans, and Louisville—paid for with municipal bonds and operated by professional doctors and nurses in contract with the government. Instead of subsidizing care at all the city's hospitals, they urged, Atlanta should build one dedicated to providing care to anyone who needed it and make it attractive enough that even those who could afford to pay would go there.

Cities across the South were having similar debates as they emerged in the decades after the war.

Many of their Northern counterparts had decades earlier decided there was wisdom in such a venture, and the hospitals they spawned had begun teaming with medical and nursing schools to provide a new array of services, including the first ambulances, which were glorified horse-drawn carriages that transported the sick and injured from homes and workplaces to the hospital for prompt treatment. New York's Bellevue Hospital, operational in one form or another since 1736, is credited with pioneering the concept of emergency transport, and the armies of the Union made great use of them during the Civil War.

In Chicago, where the Illinois general assembly assigned the care for paupers to county governments, Cook County provided food and medicine as early as 1832 in temporary hospitals and infirmaries. It ordered similar supplies for private homes that took in the poor and destitute. And students at

Rush Medical School were enlisted to provide free care.

When Chicago was hit with cholera epidemics in 1849 and again five years later, the commissioner of health prevailed upon the city to team up with Rush and use one of its buildings as a designated charity and teaching hospital. During the Civil War, Union troops used the facility as a military hospital. The city and county made a deal after the war to convert what was once a reform school into "County Hospital," an imposing brick-and-limestone building that opened for patients in 1866.

Among its modern facilities: an autopsy room. Rush Medical School set up the nation's first physician internship program there the same year. Neither the interns, nor the attending physicians who supervised their work, were paid for their services, but they gained valuable experience dealing with patients with an array of diseases and conditions.

Early Political Influence

But by this time, Chicago's political culture was already teeming with patronage and corruption, and it wasn't long before County Hospital fell into disrepair. The physicians who worked there persuaded the county to open a new hospital in 1876—this one with more than three hundred beds.

It may have been a new hospital, but it was the same Chicago, and the patronage and corruption that existed before County was created was still in place ten years later, prompting the resignation of the entire medical staff.

Ward bosses hired the replacement doctors and controlled the hospital for the next several decades. The Chicago experience of using a public charity hospital as a patronage post for politicians and their friends would unfortunately be duplicated in many cities around the country over the next century, damaging, for many of them, their public support and jeopardizing the tax base needed to keep them up and running.

But the Southern cities trying to determine whether to build charity hospitals had another factor to consider in their deliberations that their Northern counterparts seemed less troubled with: what to do with poor blacks? If indeed these new "public" hospitals were created with a mission to take in all comers, would that also include the tens of thousands of freed slaves and destitute people of color who were settling in Southern cities? And, if so, would they be treated alongside whites by the same doctors and the same nurses in integrated wards?

No doubt these and similar questions were being asked and answered around the country, but in the South they were dealt with more openly and played an integral role in the establishment of municipal hospitals. For the most part, the question in the Southern cities was easily answered by the city fathers of the time: Black patients and white patients would not be mixed. The hospitals would make services available to black patients, but in separate quarters, sometimes in separate buildings. It was an arrangement that would last decades and set a tone for future discussions about how much, and for whom, government should be required to provide health care, welfare, and other social services for the poor.

Here's how that debate played out in Atlanta in the late 1880s:

One of Henry Grady's friends, a businessman named Joseph Hirsch, took the lead in pushing Atlanta's government officials to build a charity hospital in the growing city. Grady died somewhat unexpectedly in 1888. Hirsch and others proposed the new hospital be named after him in 1890. Hirsch, proclaiming confidence that he could get individual donors and philanthropic groups to help the city finance construction, persuaded the board of aldermen to sign off on the idea that following year.

It would be a difficult effort. The issue of race—and class—was apparent almost immediately in the discussion of how much money to raise and how big the hospital should be, according to research done by Dr. Martin Moran, who wrote an exhaustive history of Grady Memorial Hospital.

The city commission that Hirsch put together had a construction committee that faced a hard question: build a hospital in stages so that it could be paid for easier and grow with the city over time, or build a hospital that would cost more initially but be able to handle Atlanta's pressing need for indigent medical care immediately upon opening.

The city took the slow-growth approach, which had been recommended by an earlier planning committee even before Grady's death. The cost of a large facility was too prohibitive, given the city's misgivings about financing a charity hospital in the first place. But there was also another reason: None of the plans that had been talked about envisioned a hospital that would treat whites and blacks in the same facility. The new hospital might open that way, but as it grew, the races would eventually be treated in separate facilities.

For the city as a whole, it was a shortsighted decision. Atlanta was growing fast. The hospital would need to double its initial capacity within ten years to keep up the ratio of beds-to-population that had become accepted around the country in 1890. But if one excluded black population growth from the equation, the plans for the new hospital seemed more than adequate, the city leaders decided.

Indeed, in the original plans for the hospital, the wards for blacks were considered a temporary solution. Builders of the hospital envisioned a separate facility for blacks a few years later, eventually turning the once black-only wards over to poor whites. Moreover, the planners said, the administrative floors of the facility could be converted to a fifteen-bed ward for the private-pay patients of the doctors who staffed it.

Dr. Moran concluded from his research that from the outset, the new hospital was supposed to be for whites only. Later, if the city could afford it, there could be two charity hospitals—one for whites and one for blacks. (It would stay that way for at least eight decades.)

Hirsch was still having a hard time raising private money to help finance the endeavor. One of the civic leaders helping Hirsch pointed out that the city's philanthropic base was already being routinely tapped for funds for the other hospitals and social services.

Plus, many were asking why they should be contributing additional money to a public hospital being paid for by the city using the hard-earned tax money already collected from them. More than one businessman pointed out that it wasn't wise to try to get money from wealthy city residents who would probably never set foot in a hospital chartered as a charitable mission to the poor. It would not be the last time that public hospital advocates would hear that complaint, in Atlanta or elsewhere.

Nevertheless, the city council and Mayor William Hemphill on August 3, 1891, approved an ordinance "pledging the city accept and sustain the Grady Hospital when completed." Section two of the ordinance also pledged the city would "maintain" the hospital. But the council struck the last four words that would have defined Grady "as a public charity," an indication of the misgivings of the city's elected leadership that the hospital could become a drain on the municipal purse.

Two months later the organizing committee for the hospital was back before the mayor and council in need of money to complete the facility.

By the time the one-hundred-bed Henry W. Grady Memorial Hospital opened its doors on May 25, 1892, Hirsch had cobbled together an impressive $104,000, about half of which came directly from city coffers. Still, it wasn't quite enough to fully equip the facility. Doctors would later complain about not having the necessary tools for surgery. But it was open, and there was room to grow.

That first day, the hospital admitted Allen Kimball, a railroad employee, who was injured on the job. Kimball later left the railroad to work at Grady, first as an orderly and then as ambulance driver. He was employed by the hospital up until the time of his death in 1931.

Grady's first patient was a black man.

2
MEDICINE AND SCIENCE

You may know him mostly as a character out of cowboy fiction, but the traveling salesman who pushed snake oils, herbal potions, and other supposedly healthful tonics was a very real fixture of life in nineteenth-century America.

Think of these colorful hucksters as the first promoters of direct-to-consumer drugs.

After all, they had almost as much credibility as physicians. And even when there was a doctor in town, the skill set he brought to his patient's bedside was largely limited to helping nature do the healing, not unlike the tonic salesman. At best, a doctor's scope of therapy included releasing toxins from the body by withdrawing blood, or pumping it with herbal mixtures carried from his home pharmacy. Perhaps with advanced training, he might be able to amputate a gangrenous limb or remove a growth of unknown origin. But there was considerable pain involved with that, not to mention the high risk of infection.

So it was in Jefferson, Georgia, in 1841, two days' ride from Atlanta and a day from Athens, when Crawford W. Long took over the medical practice of a local physician. Long was the son of a wealthy merchant and plantation owner. (He was also the cousin of the famed gambler John Henry "Doc" Holliday, who became a very real character in cowboy nonfiction.)

As a brilliant young man, Crawford Long graduated at an early age from the University of Georgia and went to Lexington, Kentucky, to study medicine at Transylvania College, where one of his instructors was Benjamin Dudley, a surgeon. Dudley had begun experimenting with alcohol concoctions, cannabis, hypnotism, and other mind-numbing methods to relieve patients from pain while under the knife. The experiments seemed to make the patients relax prior to surgery, but it was clear they were still in pain during surgery, Long recalled later.

Armed with a medical degree from the University of Pennsylvania that included a surgical residency, the newly trained physician went about the first months of his practice in Jefferson doing occasional operations on tumors and diseased tissue, delivering babies, and prescribing naturopathic remedies for fevers and seizures.

Still, he remained fascinated by Dudley's experiments and the traveling salesmen who would show up in Kentucky with diethyl ether and nitrous oxide, something they promoted to crowds as "laughing gas." Not only did these gases have entertainment value, both could be used against aches and pains, the itinerant salesmen said. Indeed, Long recalled that while in Philadelphia, the young socialites around him at elite parties would inhale ether gas to induce euphoria. While under the influence, some would fall or run into objects without feeling any pain—at least until the gas wore off.

A year or so after opening his practice, Long scheduled surgery in Jefferson for a young man who had a large tumor on his neck. He decided, rather than watch his patient writhe in pain during the procedure, he would experiment with sulfuric ether, a more potent gas than its diethyl cousin, to put his patient to sleep. The patient agreed.

It seemed to work. The patient recalled no pain during the surgery. In fact, he wasn't even sure he had surgery, other than the obvious stitches in his neck. Long used the ether on other surgical patients and began routinely to use it on women who were experiencing very hard labor and deliveries.

While the young physician kept copious notes and records of his experiments, he didn't publish them anywhere. But residents of Jefferson certainly heard about them, yet not everyone was pleased. Some accused him of witchcraft. Pain was there to cleanse the body as well as the soul, they told him.

Long was having none of that. Needless pain should not have to be endured. While he agreed with his Hippocratic oath that physicians should first do no harm, if the treatment they prescribed caused pain, they should do everything in their power to minimize it. He continued to experiment with a variety of forms of "etherization." Others around the country were experimenting as well.

The first record of ether as an anesthetic didn't appear in medical literature until 1846, even though some dentists had been using nitrous oxide and diethyl ether, with limited success, for several years before that. In an editorial in the journal *Medical Examiner*, William Morton, a Boston dentist, claimed to use sulfuric ether successfully on patients facing tooth extractions. That same year he publicly demonstrated how the gas worked on a surgical patient. By 1847 more cases of successful use of ether as anesthesia were being published in other medical journals.

It was then that Long finally decided to let the world know that he had been using sulfuric ether with surgery and childbirth patients for more than five years and with amazing success. He produced detailed records and affidavits from dozens of patients and presented them at a conference at the Medical College of Georgia. The *Southern Medical and Surgical Journal* printed his case studies in 1849, but by then, several others had already claimed the title as the physician who discovered surgical anesthesia. It would be years before surgical societies, after carefully studying his notes, officially credited Crawford W. Long as the founder of modern surgical anesthesia.

It didn't really matter to Long who got the recognition. What was more important, he said, was that modern medicine had crossed a major threshold, the ability to conquer pain.

By the outbreak of the Civil War, anesthesia had become a lifesaver in the battlefield. (Depictions of whiskey-as-anesthesia during the Civil War battlefields are largely a myth, most medical historians have concluded.) Moreover, physicians were finally making progress against infections—a mortality threat equal to the surgery itself—in the military hospitals of both armies.

They tried a bit of everything, including sterilizing surgical equipment, no easy chore under battlefield conditions. In 1863 at Lynchburg's General Hospital, surgeon John J. Terrell began to pack wounds with lint, not just to stanch bleeding, but also to keep air out. It was a crude but effective innovation.

The Science That Made Hospitals Flourish

Modern germ theory leapt forward two years later in Scotland. Joseph Lister, building on the science of Louis Pasteur and others who determined microorganisms could be transmitted through the air, began to clean the wounds of his surgical patients with carbolic acid and soak the dressings he used on them in antiseptic liquid. His records showed the death rate from infection after surgery plummeted from nearly 50 percent to about 15 percent over a five-year span. Within a decade, his methods would become the standard for surgical care.

Back in the States, surgical patients went to new "general pavilion" hospitals, where there was better ventilation, instead of the cramped, converted rooming houses that were passing as hospitals before the war. Orthopedics became a medical specialty. And, while surviving patients and their families initially complained that military surgeons were too quick to amputate shattered limbs during the war, most eventually came to agree that their chances of survival without surgery would have been next to nothing. Many were fitted with prosthetic limbs that replaced wooden pegs and allowed for more mobility.

Surgery that cures had arrived. Science was replacing snake oil.

But the surgeons would need a place to operate and for their patients to recover. More importantly, they also recognized the need for a place to work together and share news of new procedures and infection control techniques.

By the 1880s, with anesthesia and aseptic conditions for the surgical patient well established, the leaders of almost every big city in the United States began clamoring for hospitals. One government survey showed that in 1873, there were fewer than two hundred hospitals nationwide. By 1910 there would be four thousand.

At the same time, a new generation of physicians was raising esteem for the medical profession and providing hope for the future. It only made sense to connect the training of those new physicians to the new hospitals.

That marriage—public hospitals that rely on physicians in training, and medical schools that need to provide hands-on instruction beyond the classroom—remains the model for American medical education today.

With origins that trace to 1876, the Association of American Medical Colleges now represents more than 150 medical schools in the United States and Canada, 400 teaching hospitals, and 51 Veterans Affairs medical centers. Those institutions employ 148,000 faculty members and 115,000 resident physicians and provide the instruction for more than 80,000 medical students.

While the payment structure for teaching physicians was to get incredibly complicated many years later, in the 1880s it was relatively simple. In general, the hospitals paid the medical school faculty nothing, or next to it, but the physicians were at liberty to get what compensation they could from the patients they treated. Thus, wealthy and middle-class patients were often admitted as well as the indigent, although almost always in separate wards and rarely sharing the same bed linens.

The medical schools concentrated instead on renewed efforts to professionalize medicine even more by insisting on academic standards and a much more rigorous program of instruction. They did this through the control of societies that licensed physicians.

The Medical School Model

It was a major departure from the disorganized medical education system that had been in place for decades in the United States. At one point the country had several hundred medical "schools"—a loose use of the term since it wasn't even necessary to have a high school diploma to gain entrance to some of them.

The best were linked in some way to established universities, even if they maintained separate governance. They insisted that their applicants demonstrate competency in Latin and mathematics. They offered a curriculum of prescribed lectures and, after serving some form of apprenticeship, awarded medical degrees.

Many of the rest, as Abraham Flexner described them in his famous 1910 summary of American medical education in the previous century, were profit-driven enterprises "money making in spirit and object." Chairmanships and faculty appointments were bought and sold, and no prospective student was turned down if he could pay his fees or sign a note.

If a hall could be cheaply rented, and if corpses were made available for dissection and enough bones assembled to make a skeleton, Flexner reported, a medical school could easily be established. There were forty-three of them in New York alone, twenty in Cincinnati, and ten in Louisville. They were doing little more than teaching anatomy, getting cheap labor through forced apprenticeships, and charging their students for the privilege.

Knowledge about advances in medicine was not widely shared in the American schools.

The stethoscope had been used in Europe since the 1830s, but it was virtually unheard of in the States, even during the Civil War, and was not even mentioned in the catalogue of the Harvard Medical School until 1868. (The microscope did not get a mention until 1869 at Harvard.)

By the 1890s, as the number of hospitals began to grow, medical schools that were churning out less-educated doctors had begun to dwindle. No longer were two years of training—the standard for decades among the smaller and less prestigious medical schools—enough. Students would have to have six months of instruction per year for at least three years. Moreover they would be required to take coursework in pathology, chemistry, and, with the growing emphasis on infection control, histology.

When the Johns Hopkins School of Medicine in Baltimore opened in 1893, the demand it placed on would-be doctors for formal education was unprecedented: four years of study. Moreover, at Hopkins prospective students needed a college degree, establishing the concept of medical education as a field of graduate study.

Rather than using local practitioners as faculty members, the school recruited researchers and scientists, some of whom rarely saw patients and instead spent their time hovering over microscopes in laboratories. The idea was to have the students spend their first two years in the labs with them and the last two in the hospital wards treating patients.

The Hopkins model was to become the professional standard for medical education, the one that Flexner was promoting everywhere when he wrote his 1910 report.

Atlanta was still far from that standard when Grady Memorial Hospital opened with the help of $60,000 in municipal taxes in 1892.

There were at least three medical schools operating in the city at the time, with the oldest of them, Atlanta Medical College, providing most of the staff for Grady. Doctors from the Southern Medical College were still providing care to the Ivy Street Hospital. The third medical school, the Georgia College of Eclectic Medicine and Surgery, founded in Forsyth, Georgia, in 1839, moved to Atlanta in 1883.

Doctors at the Georgia College expected to be able to admit

patients, and have their students train, at the new city hospital. But the Grady administration refused, believing that two medical schools practicing there would not serve the hospital's best interest. It was the first turf war over staffing at the municipal hospital, but it wouldn't be the last.

Six years after Grady opened, the Atlanta Medical College and Southern Medical College merged. The combined school, which became the Atlanta College of Physicians and Surgeons, constituted the Grady staff.

But like many others during its time, the merged Atlanta medical school was not affiliated in any way with a college or all the resources and prospective students that colleges could provide. When the Carnegie Foundation paid for Abraham Flexner to visit and evaluate the nation's medical schools, Flexner found the College of Physicians and Surgeons to be well equipped and its work at Grady to be worthy, if not as extensive as it could be. Flexner suggested that, for the benefit of the college and Grady, the medical school become a department of the University of Georgia.

The Medical College of Georgia in Augusta had by that time long been established as the leading medical school in the state, and it had the most rigorous curriculum of study. If any school were to be affiliated with the University of Georgia, it would be MCG. The reluctance to connect itself to a university may have been caused by the University of South Carolina's rejection of the Georgia medical school's proposed affiliation years earlier. (The South Carolina university, in Columbia, was closer to Augusta than UGA in Athens.)

Whatever the reason, Flexner's suggestion for Atlanta did not go very far. There was no university in the city large enough to support a medical department. It would have to wait for several more years before a split between the Methodist Episcopal Church, South and the board of Vanderbilt University in Nashville led to the formation of Emory University in Atlanta.

By the turn of the century, Atlanta's hospitals and medical

schools were busy, enough so that like many other US cities, private philanthropies and church organizations began to think about establishing their own institutions. On Thanksgiving Day in 1901, a Baptist preacher and physician, Len G. Broughton, opened a five-bed infirmary out of a rented house near his Atlanta church. Within a decade it had grown out of the house and into a seventy-five-bed facility. Broughton hired the doctors and created a nursing school to staff it.

The opening of other hospitals raised once again the issue of caring for the poor.

Scientific Charity

Since the end of the Civil War, the principles of "scientific charity"—described by hospital historian Rosemary Stevens, as promoting "self-help rather than handouts, private efforts over those of the government and paternalism rather than egalitarianism"—were held fast by most Americans.

Hospital officials assumed patients would pay their bills whenever possible. In so doing, they would avoid condemning their patients to indigence and failure, they convinced themselves.

Unlike other countries, there would be no movement toward socialism in the United States. Instead, private charity, voluntarily given, would suffice when it came to health care. And while there may have been public hospitals built with tax dollars and receiving public monies for the services they provided, there was still a long tradition of subsidizing care for truly indigent patients in private institutions, usually in the form of a modest per diem payment. In Atlanta, that meant Grady's ability to grow and expand through local taxes was reined in by the amount the other hospitals needed to get from the city for their subsidies.

The United States roundly rejected the British concept of

"voluntary" hospitals—places where health care was entirely paid for with charitable donations. Instead, the American hospital system was evolving into hybrid institutions that had paying customers, philanthropic and religious backing, some small level of government support, and, if it could be afforded, free care for those who couldn't pay for it.

But spreading that charity to multiple levels of health care in big cities proved difficult at a time when new technologies such the X-ray machine, among other innovations, were making the cost of diagnostic care almost as expensive as treatment.

Moreover, by 1910, most physicians had changed the decades-old business model that the care they provided inside of a hospital should be free. Their practices had moved from seeing the vast majority of patients in offices, or the patient's home, to inside a hospital where they had access to laboratories and other necessities. About this same time, competition among hospitals for the most modern facilities, best-trained physicians, and patients who could pay their bills became intense.

Public and private hospitals reacted to the changed climate quite differently.

At the elite, private hospitals, wealthy patrons could easily pay the price of admission for themselves. Individual donors often sponsored indigent patients, which usually meant the patient had to demonstrate some high moral, or religious, standard. The medical staff at these hospitals was controlled by a handful of doctors—some of whom might have partial ownership in the hospital itself—and they could limit the nonpaying patients by allowing admitting privileges only to doctors who, like themselves, did not routinely treat indigent patients.

Physicians with religious and ethnic backgrounds in many parts of the country were often excluded from the staff of elite hospitals. If there was not a hospital in town sponsored by their own denomination or faith community, Roman Catholic and Jewish physicians were more likely to find their medical home in public hospitals.

Those same public hospitals in many big cities existed heavily through patronage (County General in Chicago being the most well known). Construction and equipment contracts, nonmedical staffing, and other capital and operations expenses went to friends and relatives of the politicians who controlled their budgets. Physicians and reformers urged them to be more like private hospitals. Still, although frequently corrupt, the urban political machines paid more attention to lower-class residents who needed the hospital and had no other place to go.

Despite some obvious shortcomings—there was no maternity ward or provisions to take care of children, and surgeons were required to provide their own instruments—Grady survived its first two decades of existence without too much turmoil. Hospital administrators were back before the city council several times asking for more money, but rarely getting it. City officials meanwhile complained that the hospital wasn't doing enough to collect money from patients who could afford to pay, all of which was supposed to go back to the city treasury.

There were rumblings, too, that the decision to make Grady a charity hospital for indigents would eventually bankrupt the city. Whenever there was financial turmoil in the city budget, Grady became a target for cuts, not unlike what happens today at the state and local level.

Despite the conflicts, when Atlanta voters were asked in 1910 to approve a $100,000 bond issue to expand the hospital, they overwhelmingly approved. The outcome was anything but a profile in progressivism.

"The Gradys"

Two years later a new building opened next to the original, with all of its 110 beds set aside for white patients. (Thus was fulfilled the plan discussed twenty years earlier that eventually there would be two Grady hospitals: one for whites and one for blacks.) Indeed, local residents called the new building White Grady; the older hospital, they dubbed Black Grady. In a city that still wasn't certain it could maintain a charity hospital, the 1910 money that flowed from the bond issue allowed blacks and whites finally to be treated separately. No doubt that fact contributed to the referendum's success.

Still, neither hospital had facilities to treat infectious diseases such as measles and meningitis. The only isolation ward was used for patients with sexually transmitted diseases. Black Grady still had no maternity ward, leaving black women in the city to deliver their babies at home, or on the street. While there was now a separate hospital for whites only, it wasn't well equipped, and it was constantly overcrowded with patients who could not afford to pay for their care.

Not surprisingly, white patients with money went elsewhere.

The Baptist Hospital had grown to over a hundred beds. Presbyterian Hospital was operating on Central Place in downtown Atlanta near the site of one of the city's largest churches. Seventh Day Adventists had a hospital. There were private sanatoriums opening in the city, one of them owned by two local physicians who named it Piedmont, after the plateau in the eastern United States that runs between the coast and the Appalachian Mountains. It would become the forerunner of one of the city's largest private hospitals. And, of course, the Sisters of Mercy still had St. Joseph's, the city's first hospital that started from humble beginnings in 1880.

Grady was in competition with these facilities and others, not just for patients, but more importantly for public funds. It was quickly gaining a reputation as a poor people's hospital. Once again, as they had done twenty years earlier, the city's economic boosters tried to intervene. This time they were too ambitious.

They offered up another bond issue in 1914, this one designed to modernize the facilities within the two hospitals, eliminating, for instance, the crowded waiting areas where infectious diseases could easily be transmitted. They asked for $750,000 in bonds. While the majority of city voters approved the bond issue, it took two-thirds approval to pass. They didn't meet that demand.

Clearly, there was a limit to what voters would go for when it comes to charity care for the poor.

When business and labor leaders visited the hospital a few years later, they saw cots full of patients lining the corridors of a very overcrowded Black Grady. In White Grady they found children with whooping cough and typhoid fever sharing rooms with adults.

The hospital's ambulance service, once its pride and joy, was making on average eighteen runs a day. But because of money concerns, physicians on call were reluctant to dispatch ambulances to the poorer parts of town, fearing that they would bring in too many indigent patients who would crowd paying patients out of precious bed space. Records showed that one patient hurt in a streetcar accident was turned away because physicians could not determine if the streetcar company's insurance would cover the injured man's bills.

It may have been the first recorded incidence of trauma diversion in Atlanta, a complaint Grady's current ER team often hears from ambulance crews about their competitors' refusing to take emergency cases.

The labor and business leaders joined Grady's board of trustees and administrators to demand more operational support from the city. They were turned away.

Martin Moran, in his history of Grady, offers an incident that took place a few years earlier that typified the turmoil that always seemed to surround Grady in Atlanta—then and now.

About the time the horseless carriage arrived on the scene, Grady's oat-eating horses that powered the hospital's ambulance service were nearing their life-span. Rather than replacing them with four-legged animals, the hospital administrator suggested a fleet of motorized vehicles. Grady should have the most up-to-date medical transport system, the hospital argued. But the city said the hospital would have to find a way to pay for it on its own.

It took a few years, but the hospital's trustees finally cobbled together $2,800 to purchase a 32-horsepower ambulance. It didn't have enough money yet to get insurance for it.

On one of its early runs, the new ambulance stalled astride railroad tracks in the Kirkwood area of east Atlanta. When a train plowed into it, the ambulance was rendered out of commission. Without insurance to pay for repairs, Grady would have to return to the horse-drawn ambulances. Had it not been for the donation of a motorized hearse from an Atlanta funeral-home owner, the era of mechanized ambulances at Grady may have had to wait several more years.

The original ambulance was eventually repaired and the donated hearse returned to the funeral home.

3

MEDICINE BECOMES
MORE ADVANCED, MORE AVAILABLE—
AND UNAFFORDABLE

If there is a single turning point in the complicated narrative about how America provides for health care, it wasn't the creation of Medicare and Medicaid in the 1960s, as many would presume. It took place a hundred years ago, before, during, and after World War I.

Many of the central players in the ongoing drama have retained their ideological roles; some new characters have come and gone, while still others have flipped sides altogether. But the ideological skirmish—indeed some of the very dialogue— has remained remarkably consistent.

A century later, despite the existence of Medicare and Medicaid, and a more recent iteration, the 2010 Affordable Care Act, no consensus in this uniquely American intrafamily squabble about how best to care for the poor has emerged.

Understanding what happened, or more accurately didn't happen, one hundred years ago requires a broader look at how medical care was paid for in Western Europe around the time the United States began to take its place among world powers. With the remarkable scientific advancements in that same era, medicine in the United States was swiftly moving from simply treating disease to curing it and, where the resources were available, even preventing it.

In major cities around the country, university-based medical schools were attracting well-educated graduates whose formal training was now more advanced than ever. The faculty members of those medical schools practiced with their student-physicians trailing behind them on daily rounds inside the wards of large hospitals. Their laboratory-based colleagues peered through increasingly sophisticated equipment cultivating, identifying, and labeling microbes in basement rooms of those same hospitals. The symbiotic relationship among basic science, advances in clinical care, and the "teaching hospital" was being firmly established.

DOCTORS IN TRAINING AND HOW THEY GET PAID

If you have ever been a patient at a teaching hospital, you've probably wondered who is paying for all these doctors who are constantly coming in and out of your room. The answer is complicated, and it is one of the most confusing aspects of public hospital financing.

The affiliation many public hospitals share with medical schools is one of the major differences between them and their nonprofit and community hospital competitors. Almost all hospitals pay a handful of staff physicians to be in the emergency department, or to watch over the patients admitted by private community physicians who have "privileges" at the hospital.

But teaching hospitals have "resident staff"—meaning a corps of doctors housed there 24/7 to do anything that is needed. Usually these are recent medical school graduates in their first few years of practice. They are sometimes called "house staff" or "interns." In large hospitals they can number in the hundreds.

The residents work under the direction of "attending" physicians, medical school faculty members who are ultimately responsible for a patient's care. The resident staff rotates around the hospital during their years of training so they can be exposed to many different medical specialties. After their residency, some choose a specialty and get another year or two of training in that department as a "fellow."

Patients often find residents gathered around their bed—in a time-honored teaching tool, called "rounds," where they discuss the patient's diagnosis and treatment plans with an attending physician or fellow.

Attending physicians can bill separately for their services, often through a clinical foundation at the medical school where they teach. (This allows the foundation to write off some of the unpaid bills of public hospital patients.) But who pays the residents?

That would be Medicare.

Since it was created in 1965, Medicare's Graduate Medical Education program has provided much of the funding for the clinical training and hospital experience new doctors need to enter independent practice. Teaching hospitals train more than 100,000 medical and dental residents each year, according to the American Hospital Association.

Medicare pays for this two ways. It provides a flat rate to teaching hospitals that is supposed to cover the cost of educating residents, as well as salaries and benefits for them and their supervising faculty members. The rate is set by an incredibly arcane formula going back to 1984. The number of residents the hospital employs is multiplied by, among other things, the ratio of Medicare patient days to total inpatient days at the hospital. It also compensates teaching hospitals for some indirect costs, including additional equipment they may need for education purposes.

The bottom line is that Medicare pays teaching hospitals more for services provided to Medicare patients than it does to nonteaching hospitals. Medicaid fees for these hospitals are also adjusted upward too, but not as much since states have to chip in for their share of Medicaid costs. It should be noted here that private insurance plans typically do not build in any additional payment for patients at teaching hospitals. This is another reason public hospitals have a hard time competing with private hospitals for private insurance contracts. Because of resident staff, their costs are much higher.

How that additional Medicare and Medicaid revenue is divided up depends on the contract between the hospital and the medical schools. Disputes are not uncommon. The issue is compounded when more than one medical school is involved, not just with reimbursements but in determining how many resident "slots" each school is allowed.

One group that is perpetually unhappy about it are the medical residents themselves, who often feel financially abused by the system.

Writing in *Slate* magazine in 2014, Jacob Sunshine, then a resident and president of the house staff association at the University of Washington, complained that wages for residents are outrageously low compared to what hospitals are getting for the services they provide. An emergency room nurse practitioner gets $30 to $50 an hour, he said, but the resident staff in the same ER who are required to treat patients with far more acute injuries and conditions get about a third of the hourly rate compared to nurses.

Wages paid to medical residents have not come close to matching the rising cost of medical education, Sunshine said, with many recent graduates now owing more than $200,000 in student loans.

American medicine was thriving at many levels. But for many Americans, it was becoming unaffordable. No longer was the high cost of medicine a problem just for the poor. Working-class families now worried about it, and for good reason.

The concept of providing insurance to offset the high cost of illness and injury had its roots in Europe and even, to a lesser degree, in the United States many years earlier, as a hedge against lost productivity and wages in the workplace. Indeed, Georgia—now seen as the champion of a nonunionized, right-to-work business climate—was among the first states, in 1855, to pass legislation allowing employees to sue their bosses for on-the-job injuries. The proviso, of course, was that they could prove employer negligence was the cause.

While employees may have had the right to do so, suing for lost wages on the job wasn't an effective way to protect their incomes, let alone help them pay medical bills.

It was Germany that first recognized a healthy workforce and a thriving industrial economy were linked. It even gave the concept a name: "social efficiency."

Rather than trying each individual case of injury or sickness in the workplace through litigation, the central government would establish a compensation fund that workers could tap while they were away from the job. Depending on how the program was set up, the "workmen's compensation" plan would pay for a portion of lost wages or some of the costs of medical care (or, under a few plans, both). There were a variety of mechanisms used to pay for establishing these compensation plans, but most involved some combination of a government subsidy, a tax on employers, and, in many cases, a payroll tax on workers.

Other European countries tried similar plans to ensure their workers stable incomes and maintain competitiveness in the growing world marketplace at the time. Workers in high-risk industries and guild members in trades and professions formed associations, sometimes with the agreement of the government, to subsidize what became known as "mutual benefit societies."

It's important to remember that the primary goal of all these programs—from the foundry workers in Germany to the guild workers, artisans, and tradesmen in Sweden and France—was to ensure workers against lost wages when they were not on the job. Paying for the medical expenses of whatever sickness or injury befell them was still largely up to the worker.

That began to change in Europe from 1880 to 1910 when the concept of workmen's compensation morphed into compulsory sickness insurance—the key word being *compulsory*.

In the Western democracies of the Continent, the centuries-old reliance on charity and religious societies to provide for the sick and the poor no longer seemed to work for a rapidly growing, industrialized population.

Paternalism in the form of government subsidies to these groups, occasional cash assistance for individuals through local "poor relief" programs, and government-owned almshouses were thought to be holding back opportunity for growth and commerce. Many asked whether it might not be better to create a social insurance system that provided the right to certain benefits such as lost wages, health care, and even funeral expenses rather than merely subsidizing workers through charity.

Medicine and Maintaining Empires

It wasn't always altruism that motivated the discussion or the political decisions made by European leaders at the time.

In a unified Germany, Otto von Bismarck faced considerable pressure from Social Democrats to fully integrate workers into an expanded social welfare system. Business and military leaders in Great Britain thought social insurance would increase productivity, reduce class resentment, and create a healthier workforce and a stronger army. In defense of the social insurance movement, Prime Minister Lloyd George was famously quoted as saying, "You cannot maintain an A-1 empire with a C-3 population."

Whatever the reasoning, a new principle in how to pay for health care was being created on that side of the Atlantic—a principle that was not lost on business and government leaders in the States, but not at all embraced by them either.

Governments in Europe moved to compel individuals, and the employers they worked for, to make contributions for the social welfare of the whole nation. It was not unlike the concept of compulsory education that began to take root during the same time. If children had a right to a public education, the belief held, did they not also have an obligation to attend school? By the turn of the twentieth century, the answer in Europe was increasingly yes. Compulsory sickness insurance took its place next to compulsory education. Those countries have not wavered much from this basic tenet of social welfare since then.

Not so across the Atlantic. Then, or even now.

Students of American history understand that during this same time, the federal government was anything but a strong organizer of social policy in the States. In the turmoil of the post–Civil War era—indeed after the one trauma that solidified the dominance of a national government over a collection of states—the federal government nonetheless was loathe to impose further rules and regulations on the cost of doing business in the States in the last half of the 1800s.

Medicine was advancing at a rapid pace; hospitals were being built in unprecedented numbers; and public health issues arose that were clearly connected to the new industrialized and urbanized population base. Yet no one in Congress or the White House during this time took a central role in advocating how health care was to be delivered or paid for. There was no Otto von Bismarck or Lloyd George leading, much less dictating, as they did in Europe, the discussion here.

In the post–Civil War era, many states moved forward with workmen's compensation plans of their own, but those plans were still largely limited to cash benefits to make up for lost wages. Some American employers teamed up with workers to offer sickness insurance that went beyond lost wages, but it was still largely limited to medical care of injuries and sickness that could be conclusively connected to the workplace.

By 1910, with the cost of medicine rising, many workmen's compensation plans—where they existed—were no longer coming close to matching the wages Americans were losing by not being on the job because of poor health or injury. Moreover, a new generation of sociologists and reformers in the country compiled dozens of surveys over the next decade that showed a clear connection between sickness and poverty. Some labor activists and academicians began to argue that a healthy workforce would create a healthier economy.

The Rise of Workmen's Comp

The numbers they compiled in their surveys were compelling.

Workers in 1919 were estimated to lose at least $600 million a year in lost wages due to sickness and injury, a sum that was greater than the nation's entire debt five years earlier. American families were spending more than $1 billion a year on medical and hospital care, a staggering figure for a people who were not used to counting into the B's (meaning billions) for anything.

Another survey of workers in New York State showed they had received $10 million worth of "free" treatment from private and public hospitals alone in 1919. Physicians were said to have provided $12 million in charity care to New Yorkers the same year.

A landmark study published by the Illinois Health Insurance Commission provided even starker numbers.

At the individual level, workmen's compensation no doubt was helpful. Lost wages from medical problems were two to four times greater for workers than the costs associated with caring for their illness or injury. But when the cost of health care for their spouses and children in Illinois were factored in, the resulting loss more than eclipsed what they were getting in workmen's compensation.

Going over the records of nearly 4,500 workers, the Illinois commission found that about 25 percent of them were sick for a week or longer every year. The missed time cost the workers and their families, on average, about $120, which represented about 14 percent of the family's annual wages. The survey further showed that, when faced with a serious illness, about one in six families would have to rely on charity care to make ends meet.

Echoing findings that still resonate nearly a hundred years later in studies identifying medical bills as the leading cause of bankruptcy, the Illinois commission in 1919 found that perhaps a third of all charity care cases in the state could be traced, not to the impoverished or indigent, but to the working Americans who simply could not afford to pay for the care their families needed to stay well.

When Germany, England, and other European nations faced similar findings decades earlier, they moved toward compulsory social insurance plans. That concept never caught hold in the States, despite the fact that buying insurance against unplanned events was not a new concept in America.

Indeed, one of the most successful sales lines in the insurance industry came in the form of "industrial life" insurance sold to many working-class families during this era. Metropolitan Life Insurance and Prudential became industry leaders in selling policies aimed at providing benefits for funeral coverage and expenses of a final illness or injury. Newspaper advertisements at the time touted how workers who purchased this type of life insurance would relieve their widows and orphans from the embarrassment of a pauper's burial for them, should they die.

To make sure families didn't fall behind on their premiums, the companies employed a cadre of individual agents who showed up at the door to collect payments, usually within a day or two of payday. Still, lapses in premiums were frequent, and many policies expired without ever paying benefits. Moreover, with all those agents collecting a fee, the administrative costs were staggering, resulting in only an average of 40 percent of benefits paid on the cost of all premiums.

Still, in 1911 Metropolitan Life, Prudential, and other insurance companies sold $183 million in industrial life plans. Advocates of compulsory insurance in the States were quick to point out that sum was about the same as the cost of the social insurance system in place in Germany that year.

So why wasn't there a similar drive for social insurance in the States?

Dozens of academics in history, economics, and medicine have produced hundreds of books and publications studying this question. Their answers are usually organized around one or more of these findings:

- The American labor movement could not agree on the idea.

- American physicians first endorsed it, but then changed their minds.

- Even though Theodore Roosevelt and his Progressive Party pushed it, he did not have the clout at that point in his storied career to make it happen, and there was no other dominant American politician to advocate for it.

- The insurance industry was solidly against it.

- And, finally, World War I happened just as the debate was being joined. The rhetoric used to generate support for US involvement in the conflict—aimed heavily at the "Prussian menace"—spilled over into easy opposition for creating anything like the social welfare system that Germany had come to represent.

But it's worth noting there was an important debate about it during this time, nonetheless, if for no other reason than to establish how the issue was framed; how political, business, labor, and medical leaders dealt with it; and how, now a century later, we still hear many of the same arguments.

The First Shot at Universal Coverage

While Great Britain was debating and enacting its social insurance plans, a group called the American Association of Labor Legislation was drafting a similar proposal in the States. A progressive group of reformers who were unfairly criticized later as anticapitalist, the AALL, drafted a bill for compulsory sickness insurance, based mostly on the British model, to present to Congress and the states.

The "Americanized" version of the legislation guaranteed coverage to all working-class families earning less than $1,200 a year. It mandated benefits to pay for the charges of physicians and nurses, hospitalization, sick pay, and maternity services. And since industrial death benefits were so popular with the working class, the new program would also pay a $50 benefit for funeral expenses.

The entire plan would be paid for with premiums paid by workers, employers, and, when needed, a subsidy by the government.

Many prominent physicians at the time endorsed the idea. The American Medical Association even passed a resolution favoring it in 1917. But it wasn't long before the nation's largest physician organization—as would happen at other critical junctures in the future—found its membership splintered on the idea.

More importantly, despite AALL having labor roots, the American Federation of Labor stood steadfast against it. The AFL argued that if compulsory health insurance became law, especially at the state level, government would be given too much power over the health of workers.

The union also worried, no doubt, that government-endorsed health insurance plans would weaken the union's role in providing social benefits for its workers. There was no real collective bargaining at the time for wages, so negotiating for social benefits was the AFL's major responsibility. (Fast-forward nearly one hundred years later, and you can hear some of the same misgivings labor leaders expressed about the role Obamacare might play in usurping collective bargaining for wages and benefits in those industries where unions remain a force.)

Perhaps the biggest threat to the insurance industry that opposed the legislation a hundred years ago was the funeral benefit. It seems strange in the modern era to think that something as minuscule as a $50 funeral benefit would get the industry in such an uproar, but it clearly did, and it awakened a sleeping giant in doing so.

Those industrial life insurance policies were money in the bank for the commercial insurance industry, so a new, government-backed benefit—collected through payroll deductions and at the same time with premiums for sickness insurance—clearly jeopardized the profitability of the companies writing them, not to mention the armies of salesmen making a living promoting the policies and collecting the premiums.

At about the time of America's entry to the Great War, newspaper and magazine articles began appearing prominently calling out Germany's role in promoting "socialist insurance" and linking the concept with the rise of socialist parties in Europe. Such ideas were inconsistent with American values, the thought leaders of the time said.

In America, we can take care of our own. Through hard work, charity at the church, parish, and synagogue, affiliation with worker unions and the beneficence of enlightened employers, the United States need not sink to the level of demanding its people purchase sickness insurance.

But with the Red Scare and the rise of Russian and Eastern European Bolshevism after the war—despite the demonstrable need for help seen in the surveys of workers around the country at the time—the debate over how to make health care more affordable through government-backed health insurance was effectively over. It would not come up again until Franklin D. Roosevelt was president, and then it would be subjugated to a more palatable goal of providing income security for the elderly.

A Stronger Marriage between Hospitals and Medical Schools

While the debate over compulsory insurance exhausted itself after World War I, there was steady movement toward advanced medical education and the implementation of clinical science in the wards of American hospitals. Much of that work took place in public hospitals that solidified their relationships with medical schools and earned them reputations as the go-to place for the latest treatments and procedures.

The symbiosis between the large urban hospital and academia provided an ideal setting to broaden the education and experience of a new generation of physicians before they went into practice for themselves. General hospitals attracted patients afflicted with a wide assortment of maladies, ranging from chronic conditions such as hypertension and diabetes to exotic infections contracted in faraway places and brought to American shores by immigrants and travelers.

Hospitals began to segregate patients by their conditions:

surgical patents occupying one floor, maternity and delivery on another, infectious diseases farther away from the general population and isolated in wards with a dedicated doctor and nursing staff.

Laboratories, usually in the basements and lower floors, were created to quickly determine what pathogens might be causing a patient's unknown illness. Radiology equipment, the technology of which seemed to be improving each year, allowed physicians to see shadows inside patients' bodies to help them determine what should, and should not, be there.

The medical schools constituted the "house staff" for many of these hospitals. Full faculty members could see any patient who walked through the doors, as well as admitting patients from their own practice. The next tier of physicians worked full time in the hospital, "attending" patients from one room to the next and from ward to ward, while others specialized in certain diseases. And trailing behind the attending staff, taking it all in and sometimes performing tests and procedures themselves, were students who had completed their anatomy, chemistry, biology, and other classroom work during the first two years of medical school and were now getting valuable hands-on experience as physicians.

This formula for graduate medical education—one that still largely exists today—became a standard at the same time large municipal hospitals and the medical schools associated with them were catapulting clinical, emergency, and critical care into a new era.

At Cook County Hospital in Chicago, the first blood bank for use in surgery was opened in the mid-1930s, following the discovery of ways to safely store blood. Patients who "bled out" during risky surgery almost always died or were permanently harmed. With blood at the standby, surgical risk was significantly reduced.

Manipulating blood pressure, and discovering other ways to reduce bleeding, allowed surgeons at Charity Hospital in New

Orleans to perfect a procedure for treating life-threatening aneurysms, where blood vessels balloon and tear open unexpectedly.

And there was remarkable progress in the battle against death and disability due to trauma and injury.

Once the exclusive purview of military surgeons at battlefield hospitals, trauma care moved into the civilian sector in a big way in the 1930s. The medical staff of Los Angeles General Hospital was pressed into service treating blunt trauma and other injuries, with remarkable success, after a major earthquake rocked Southern California in 1933. Cook County and San Francisco General hospitals established the first formal trauma units in American hospitals about this same time.

Other general hospitals quickly followed suit, so much so that local ambulance crews began to transport severely injured patients past the emergency rooms of private hospitals to take them directly to the area's general hospital.

Faculty members kept detailed notes on their patients and published studies in peer-reviewed journals. New rounds of clinical experimentation with drugs and procedures—this time using patients instead of laboratory animals—commenced, often with mixed results. (It would be a few years before strict standards of ethics of human experimentation would be created.)

Soon, the marriage between academic medicine and the large, urban hospital was officially consummated.

The Emory-Grady Connection Is Established

In Atlanta, Grady Memorial Hospital, not yet twenty-five years old, found a new courtship developing with Emory University, whose early leaders decided they would build a university encompassing not just a liberal arts undergraduate program, but professional schools as well.

Emory moved quickly to establish a presence for its medical school students and professors at Grady, which by then had begun to lose many of its connections to the older and less prestigious (at least in terms of admission requirements) medical schools in Atlanta. Still, city leaders and hospital administrators didn't think it wise to turn over control of the medical staff to the upstart school. So they came up with another idea.

Emory could have Black Grady.

The segregated public hospital—where white patients were cared for in the newest building, black patients in the oldest and least equipped—could use the help that Emory offered. Plus, once Emory took on responsibility for patient care at the black hospital in 1921, the medical staff at White Grady reorganized and formed what amounted to a new medical school, the Atlanta Graduate School of Physicians and Surgeons (AGS). When a new, modern clinic opened at White Grady in 1924, the new school ran the show.

AGS wasn't as much a medical school as it was a for-profit practice of the four physicians who owned it, ran it, and hired young physicians just out of medical school to work for them. Grady's administrators and the city council complained that they were left out of the decision-making about what was happening at White Grady.

It wasn't public officials who pushed back most effectively against the school and its administrators; it was their students and the associated medical staff. They battled for nearly two years with work stoppages and other tactics, forcing the school to concede more power to both the hospital and the associated physicians who worked there. Still, distrust lingered among the doctors serving White Grady.

Meanwhile Emory was improving Black Grady with its own money. For more than a decade, the equipment and facilities at Black Grady had steadily deteriorated—the result of a city council that could never seem to find the money to improve conditions there.

In the years following its affiliation with Grady, Emory at times even helped make the payroll at the black hospital—at one point putting up $30,000 in staff salaries. (Fast-forward about eighty years, as we shall see in a future chapter, Emory kept Grady solvent by essentially floating a more than $60 million debt the hospital owed it for medical services rendered.)

Patient Safety at Risk at Grady

Despite Emory's help, Black Grady was still a rat's nest, literally and figuratively. Because of the age of the hospital and lack of maintenance, the place was overrun with cockroaches and vermin. The Emory medical staff complained that rats in the nursery had bitten several newborns. Minutes of a medical staff meeting in April of 1925 reflect a report that a premature newborn in the nursery may have died as the result of a rat bite.

Five years later, rats apparently chewed through insulation surrounding the wiring in the radiology lab, sparking a fire, which in turn caused canisters of X-ray film to explode and spread noxious gas through the building. No one was seriously hurt, but fifteen patients had to be evacuated through the windows.

For that matter, White Grady was nothing to shout about. It wasn't nearly as advanced as other teaching hospitals around the country at this time. Infectious disease patients shared space with postsurgery patients. Measles and chicken pox outbreaks in the pediatric ward would force the unit to be quarantined, and no child could enter or exit until the outbreak had been controlled.

By 1930 there was a significant movement toward turning control of the medical staffs of both the black and white hospitals over to Emory.

One of the community leaders who opposed the idea was the Reverend Leonard Broughton, pastor of the Baptist

Tabernacle and a physician by training. Broughton was considered a supporter of Grady even though he was founder of
Georgia Baptist Hospital a few blocks away. But when the idea
surfaced about Emory and White Grady, Broughton wanted
nothing to do with it.

The Georgia Baptist Hospital and Grady were both competing for patients who could pay the full freight for their care,
meaning, at the time, white patients. There was no real competition for black and indigent patients in Atlanta. By then, they
were already being channeled to Grady. As the city's public hospital, this was part of its mission. Competing hospitals didn't
necessarily refuse black and poor patients; they just couldn't
afford to take too many of them.

Georgia Baptist was in such a predicament. While it had
been in operation for more than twenty-five years, it was barely
breaking even. The Georgia Baptist Convention, its owner,
wanted to support Broughton and the hospital, but it had other
missions on its agenda too. If Grady siphoned away white, paying customers, Georgia Baptist might have had to close its doors.

Interestingly, Broughton's religious convictions about poor
conditions at Black Grady and the risk of abuse of patients
played perhaps an equally important role in his opposition.

He feared that if Emory took over medical care at White
Grady, it too would begin to neglect Black Grady. Even worse,
Broughton predicted, the new era of medical experimentation
would exploit black patients as human guinea pigs for treatments and procedures that, at worst, might kill them and, at
best, would ultimately benefit only whites. He roundly condemned the city's leaders and business elite for neglecting Black
Grady for all those years.

At his church one night in 1930, Broughton preached
fire and brimstone in a sermon he titled, "The Exploitation of
Atlanta's Negroes and Poor." From the pulpit he framed the
issue this way: "Shall Grady Hospital be made the experiment
station with the poor blacks and whites as the victims while

Atlanta's rich roll and fly in sumptuous luxury?" Such rhetoric would resurface during the desegregation movement and again years later when the hospital's finances and governance came under attack.

The Reverend Broughton's point of view in 1930, however, did not resound within the larger community. Moreover, there was a keen interest in Emory's desire to have more say over the entire hospital. An independent medical school, chartered as an institution of advanced learning, might remove the political patronage connected to the running of a large public hospital.

None of this, mind you, changed how health care was paid for in Atlanta in general, or at Grady in particular. All the same problems paying for medical bills that afflicted working-class people elsewhere in the country, afflicted those same people in Atlanta. If anything, those problems were more acute in Atlanta, whose impoverished population was larger than most cities in the North and Midwest at the time.

But the affiliation with Emory locked Grady into a relationship that, over time, proved mutually beneficial, even if decades later the financial relationship between the two of them remained largely a mystery to many state and local political leaders.

4

THE OLD IDEAL AND THE NEW DEAL

During the Great Depression and in the years following it, the uniquely American way of caring for the sick and the poor faced its most serious challenge. The widely held belief that the national government should play only a limited role in securing the health and welfare of its citizens—a concept that European nations decades earlier decided was socially, economically, and morally ineffective—would be debated in a way that continues to set the tone for public-policy discussions even today.

The old ideal that private organizations, religious groups, and wealthy individuals are better stewards of the poor than government could ever be was no match for the economic upheaval inflicted on the country during the Great Depression.

The earlier precept of "scientific charity" had steadily evolved over fifty years to call for government subsidies to these private benefactors, mostly in the form of small grants, courtesy of taxpayers at the local level. Those stipends helped convert almshouses for the poor in the post–Civil War era into the nation's first real hospitals. By the 1930s, there were an estimated four thousand medical facilities nationwide serving the poor and affluent alike, even if often they were in separate and anything-but-equal quarters.

Atlanta's Grady Memorial Hospital, created four decades earlier with a specific mission to serve the poor, by this time was barely scraping by, overwhelmed with patients—many of whom could not pay. Grady's construction was partially financed by city taxes, and some of its services were offset by local government subsidies. But the city's bond issues for subsequent expansions and much-needed improvements were woefully inadequate. It continued to deteriorate while newer, private hospitals sprang up around it.

That meant getting paying customers in the doors often took priority over Grady's charity mission, just so the hospital could stay afloat. That same demand to find paying patients so that vital services were still available for those who could not pay—the economic two-step we later came to call "cost shifting"—was at play in virtually every large public hospital in the United States when the stock market crashed in 1929.

Still, there was no real movement toward compulsory sickness insurance plans like those publicly financed programs adopted years earlier in Germany, Great Britain, and other European nations.

The moral hazard that underpinned the American preference for private versus government charity—the bedrock belief that instituting government-financed programs for the health and welfare of individuals would most certainly lead them to a life of dependency—remained strong even during the nation's most serious financial crisis.

This was unique to America, sociologist Paul Starr points out in his landmark book, *The Social Transformation of American Medicine*. In both Germany and England, there was initial opposition to government-financed health insurance too, but opponents did not suggest enacting it would sap the self-reliance of the citizenry. The focus instead was on how to decentralize the new systems to keep both physician societies and insurance companies happy.

Additionally, by associating the call for such a scheme in the states with the "enemy regimes" of Germany and Russia, Starr writes, the powerful opponents of an American plan made easy work of dismissing it even during the Depression years. Opponents countered that "voluntary" insurance was the American way, even though "compulsory" education—requiring children to go to school and providing tax dollars to support schools—was a well-established public policy by then.

Branding "Socialized Medicine" in the Political Arena

Compulsory insurance, opponents argued, amounted to social-ism, and they were very successful at selling that claim. Tagging universal health insurance as "socialized medicine" remains an effective diversion in public discussion of health care reform today.

In the early twentieth century, the United States created a political trap for itself from which it has yet to be released, Starr believes. He notes that the nation's history since World War I and the Great Depression has been to enact a series of incre-mental changes in health care financing. Each was designed to deal with a specific problem at the time. Each enriched the market for one major player in the health care industry or another. And each helped pacify—at least temporarily—pub-lic demand to control costs. Nevertheless, because of the com-plexity of the evolving system over the years, costs continued inexorably to mount.

"We satisfied the majority of the public," Starr said in an interview on National Public Radio. But in so doing, "we bur-ied a lot of the cost" for what consumers were really paying.

The first group to be exempted from the American dogma of self-reliance was the elderly.

By virtue of longevity (and in the 1930s policy debate, their inability to fully participate in the workforce), the elderly had earned their status as worthy recipients of the federal govern-ment's beneficence, or so many Americans were persuaded. They were entitled to a government-guaranteed pension, the nation's leadership decided, but that would have to suffice. Still, there would be no government-guaranteed health insur-ance, even for the elderly, at least not for another few decades.

Hospitals, on the other hand, would get more help during the 1930s and the time immediately before and after World War II. The purchase of voluntary insurance, usually in the form of prepaid plans offered through employers, became more commonplace. New insurance plans connected workers in specific industries, trades, and professions to specific hospitals where their major medical expenses were paid for when they needed care. With wages and earnings still suffering after the Depression, these benefits became all the more important, and hospitals came to understand that insurance companies, perhaps more so than patients, were their real customers.

No doubt these private group plans were helpful to Americans who were lucky enough to go back to work and qualify for coverage. But for American hospitals, they ushered in an era of stabilization and growth. The private insurance marketplace forced competition for insured patients between private, nonprofit hospitals and public hospitals. Not surprisingly, private hospitals fared best in this scheme.

And with the veneration of American free enterprise and competition after World War II—when the federal government once again faced the call for universal health insurance—it was also no real surprise that it chose instead to try to help by creating more hospitals and more competition.

Hospitals and the New Deal

At the height of the Great Depression, with one in four able-bodied American men unable to get work, finding a way to cushion the blow of unemployment became a compelling, and sellable, cause for social reformers. While it once placed third in the priority list of progressives, behind universal health insurance and old-age pensions, unemployment insurance was now front and center. The movement gained momentum first among the states, with about a half-dozen adopting plans.

Similarly, before the 1929 crash, there was a steady movement toward making it easier for older workers to leave their jobs to make room for younger replacements. Five states had old-age pension laws before 1932, agreeing with reformers that the elderly would need some kind of income security in their remaining years of life if they weren't working.

Combining these two ideas of old-age pensions and unemployment insurance—and finding a champion for them in Franklin D. Roosevelt—set the stage for what became the Social Security Act, the nation's most ambitious effort to date in dealing with social welfare issues of its citizens.

While FDR's Social Security triumph and his administration's public-works jobs programs are universally accepted (or condemned, depending on your point of view) as the beginning of the US welfare state, it is perhaps more important to examine how they were created, how they were paid for, and what they left out.

Despite strong advocacy from progressives and academics, FDR's Committee on Economic Security determined relatively quickly in 1934 that including any form of compulsory health insurance in the legislation would, as insiders say now, render the plan dead on arrival in Congress. Indeed, the final bill only mentioned the need for the Social Security Board to study the idea. (Even that glancing reference prompted the AMA to hold a special meeting to condemn the idea and promote instead its point of view that voluntary health insurance might work as long as local medical societies controlled payment mechanisms.)

Furthermore, conservatives in Congress tamped the benefits of unemployment insurance and old-age pensions considerably once they got ahold of Roosevelt's bill.

The financing mechanism they devised for the Social Security Act was a regressive federal payroll tax that excluded the very poor as well as those who were paid in cash, like farmers and domestic employees. When administration promoters asked that the old-age pensions in the states be required "to pay a subsistence compatible with decency and health," the language was cut from the bill at the insistence of state officials in the South. Their fear was that including the provision would be the first step toward compelling them to pay higher pensions to blacks.

The final measure did not exclude health care altogether, even if it didn't tackle the issue of insurance. As Starr has pointed out, the Social Security Act of 1935 extended the limited role of the federal government in promoting some public health programs by greatly enhancing the concept of "matching" funds. (If the states would agree to kick in some general revenue for a needed project or plan, the federal government would match or exceed it.)

Among other things, the alphabet soup of New Deal jobs programs was pressed into service to renovate hospitals and health care facilities, especially those run by state and local governments. Money in the Public Works Administration and the Works Progress Administration budgets went toward construction of psychiatric facilities around the country, as well as tuberculosis facilities in places where the lung disease remained a public health menace. (Over the years, many of these psychiatric hospitals would fall into disrepair and be the target of numerous criminal investigations of scandalous abuses of the vulnerable patients within them. The resulting furor, as we shall see in a subsequent chapter, led to the "deinstitutionalization" movement of the 1960s when thousands of mentally ill patients were released to community services unprepared to handle the severity of their conditions.)

The New Deal also included federal money to match state taxes that were being used for maternal and infant care and rehabilitation services for crippled children, as well as money for some basic public health and sanitation programs.

More importantly, the federal government would match state funding for aid to families with children under the age of sixteen. The inclusion of this last provision would become immensely important in the funding and structure of health and welfare programs for the poor in the decades to come.

But the two main components of the Social Security

Act—unemployment insurance and old-age pensions—differed in how they were administered. For one thing, unemployment insurance remained voluntary for the states. And there was some initial reluctance within the states to sign up, even though federal taxes would help finance the program.

Court Challenges to Social Security Preview What Would Come

Conservatives in Washington and in the states objected to the very idea and sued to stop it. The case wound up before the Supreme Court two years after the law was passed. But when the high court upheld the law, states quickly fell in line. Still, they retained their critical role in administering benefits at the local level, based on the belief that local officials were in a better position to determine if individuals were abusing it. This would play out exactly the same way with the creation of Medicare and Medicaid three decades later.

In contrast, the old-age pension provisions of the Social Security Act always enjoyed wider acceptance among politicians and voters, perhaps the result of the havoc caused by the Great Depression for a generation of Americans who had worked hard and whose meager savings would never be recovered. As a result, New Deal advocates and their supporters had little trouble rallying Congress to enact a dedicated payroll tax to protect the elderly from the uncertainty of the nation's free-market economy.

The pension provisions of the law, for the first time, put the federal government in the position of securing a steady flow of income for the vast majority of the nation's elderly—regardless of their economic status, their work history, or other means and abilities that had been used in their younger years to determine whether they were worthy of government help.

Most importantly, states had no real say over the pension

plan. The payroll tax, which was levied on workers and their employers, went to Washington and into a separate fund. The benefits were paid back out to recipients when they reached the qualifying age. It was as simple, and as revolutionary, as that. Nor has the concept changed much since the law was enacted in 1935.

Still, the antagonism toward the New Deal's social programs among Southern politicians was extensive, especially among Roosevelt's fellow Democrats.

Georgia Governor Eugene Talmadge welcomed the flow of dollars from Washington for road construction programs, but not for public health and welfare programs. One estimate of spending in Georgia in 1936 showed the state spent about $6 per resident on highways compared to $1 per resident on education.

As Southern historian James C. Cobb of the University of Georgia notes, state leaders throughout the South "were more than willing to let people starve on the steps of their capitols to get more highway money." As a result, public health fared much, much worse—a few pennies per year per Georgia resident during the New Deal.

Nevertheless, with more job-creating power vested in the federal government than ever before, FDR's administration found ways around the reluctant politicians to get New Deal money flowing to improve health in the states.

For example, the Civil Works Administration temporarily employed thousands in Georgia to combat the sources of typhus, hookworm, and malaria. At Grady Hospital, the federal government pumped more than $300,000 into the hospital through the CWA, the Works Progress Administration, and the Federal Emergency Relief Administration.

More significantly, the CWA included some funds to hire nurses and other nonphysicians at Grady and other hospitals where they were needed. But when Senator Richard Russell, a Georgia Democrat, heard about the plan—including a requirement that would have paid the CWA nurses more than those employed by the hospital—it was shut down in its tracks.

Hiring a few hundred folks to paint the hospital's walls was one thing, local and state politicians complained. But setting wages for new workers, putting them in competition for jobs with permanent workers, and creating an expectation of higher pay for everyone was quite another.

"Demonizing" the New Deal in the South

Because many of the New Deal jobs "had strings attached to the federal money that came with them," including minimum wages and hiring through unions where unions existed, Cobb said, the programs ran afoul of Southern politicians who were eager to keep union strength in the region suppressed.

Going back a decade or more before the Civil War, there is "a long history of Southern politicians demonizing the federal government as an agent for the North, and they sold that to lower-class whites," the UGA historian said.

When it came to job creation programs coming down from Washington, Cobb continued, "The sales pitch boiled down to warnings that these programs were geared toward training blacks for white jobs."

Still, the infusion of money from the New Deal programs helped relieve Grady temporarily from its reliance on local government to offset its considerable expenses. The Atlanta region continued to grow during the lead up to Depression years, and Grady's administrators noticed that many of its patients—about one in four—were coming from parts of Fulton County outside the city of Atlanta. They were keenly aware that Atlanta taxpayers were, in essence, subsidizing the care of non-Atlanta residents.

In 1931 they presented the Fulton County Commission a bill for the care of indigent county residents and suggested a grant of $100,000 from county taxpayers would be appropriate.

The county had been contributing $10,000 per year toward Grady's expenses but still well below the $160,000 per year in bills the hospital's administrators said Fulton residents were running up.

If the county didn't want to pay the bill, the hospital suggested an alternative—a per diem charge for Fulton County patients. That proposal got nowhere. Instead the county agreed in 1936 to pay $40,000 a year.

Interestingly, this rudimentary form of negotiating a yearly subsidy remains in place today. Every year during budget deliberations, the Fulton County Commission gets an estimate of the cost of indigent patient care from the hospital, and Grady often settles for less, while other times it is grateful for a million or two more.

In the years after the creation of Social Security and other New Deal programs, prominent liberals in Washington—notably Senator Robert F. Wagner (D–NY)—pressed FDR and his administration to return to the idea of constructing a health insurance plan along the same lines as the pension plan. And in 1938, in the middle of Roosevelt's second term, a conference brought together labor, farmers, and doctors (business was notably missing) to discuss it. The president clearly was interested, but the AMA and the insurance industry had other ideas.

For the first time, the AMA recognized that there might be a need for some kind of a plan for the "medically indigent." But whatever it was, it should be carried out at the local level with local medical societies making the decisions, the doctors said. By taking this step, the AMA said, national health insurance would not be necessary, and the risk of creating a socialized medical plan like those in Europe could be averted.

The AMA's position was little more than a talking point during the debate, but it was framed as a wiser alternative. In the end, it really didn't matter.

Elections that same year ushered in a new, more conservative Congress dedicated to reining in FDR's programs. The president backed off support for a national plan, telling supporters it might have to wait for the 1940 presidential election. Instead, he offered a program aimed at providing federal funds to construct hospitals in needy areas. That proposal died in Congress, but it would come up again ten years later when FDR's vice president succeeded him in office.

There was no more talk of compulsory health insurance in the FDR White House years. World War II loomed.

The Rise of the Blues

The New Deal money that flowed to the nation's hospitals for renovations and improvements was important, but finding a way to help patients pay for the high cost of the increasingly technologically advanced care being provided at American hospitals held the biggest challenge to their survival.

The answer would lie in the expansion of voluntary group health insurance not unlike the plans popular in the World War I era that helped workers offset their lost wages when they were sick.

About the time of the stock market crash, the vice president of Baylor University Medical School in Dallas, Justin Ford Kimball, struck upon an idea that within a few years would take the concept one important step further. Baylor had taken over the former Texas Baptist Memorial Sanitarium a few years earlier, and its medical school faculty, attending physicians, and students served as its primary staff.

If Baylor Hospital created a prepaid insurance plan and sold it to the very people who were likely to need its services, the result would be a win-win, as we would say today. The potential patient would be covered for expensive services, and the hospital would be assured of a steady stream of income and many fewer unpaid bills.

Kimball's business plan targeted Dallas teachers, especially those employed by his own university. Baylor Hospital had been running significant debt during the Depression, much of it from educators who could not pay their bills.

Kimball suggested this deal: For $6 a year, the educators could enroll in a prepaid plan that guaranteed up to twenty-one days of care in the university hospital. Remarkably, 75 percent of them signed up. Word of the plan spread quickly through Dallas. Local banks signed on. So did the daily newspaper.

Hospitals and employers around the country adopted the blueprint for prepaid hospital insurance that Kimball created in the 1930s. The American Hospital Association (AHA) took notice.

As interest among employers spread, the association moved quickly to adopt a set of standards that defined what benefits the insured should expect and what hospitals could expect to be paid for providing them. Within a few years, the AHA had successfully consolidated many of the plans and created what came to be known as the Blue Cross network. By 1938 more than one million Americans were covered by the network of nonprofit insurance plans operating mostly on the state level.

It's significant that this trend toward prepaid health insurance was started and stimulated by hospitals from the nonprofit sector. The reason was the high cost of medicine practiced in hospital settings, which was rapidly becoming unaffordable to most of the population. Similar prepaid plans for physician services between employers and "medical service bureaus" (or groups of cooperating physicians) also existed in the country, but they were limited to employees in certain high-risk industries, such as mining and timber.

For most workers, the cost of going to the doctor for simple ailments and injuries could be worked into their family budgets. It would be a generation or more before Blue Shield networks of insurance to cover physician services came into being, after federal law was changed to provide tax breaks for companies that subsidized employee insurance. And it would be 1982 before the Blues were combined into the powerhouse for health insurance they are today.

Still, this concept of hospital insurance first, doctors insurance second, has had profound consequences.

When Medicare was established in 1965, as we shall see in the next chapter, the government payment mechanism covering bills for the elderly was a trust fund covering hospital services only. Elderly patients who wanted Medicare coverage for physician services had to purchase Medicare Part B, which was paid for entirely with premiums deducted, usually, from their Social Security checks.

It wasn't as if hospitals pulled a fast one, or got to the insurance trough first. The modern hospital of the 1930s, as indeed it is today, was a medical miracle. But the services that were provided within it—then and now—were unaffordable for most people.

The presumption that physician services would stay affordable to the masses, even those covered by insurance, would be severely tested. Decades later—as EKGs, X-ray machines, laboratories, rehabilitation services, and even surgery became routine in "outpatient" settings—the different payment structures within the old Blue Cross plans and Blue Shield plans, not to mention Medicare Part A and Part B, would make it difficult to switch emphasis from acute care to primary care.

The growth of nonprofit insurance plans like Blue Cross helped stabilize the hospital market in the 1930s, especially among nonprofit hospitals. Yet it also fundamentally altered their business models, making them more aware than ever that their very existence was dependent on attracting insured patients.

Prior to the Great Depression, most of them operated with small reserves using physicians who donated their time and employing nurses and other personnel working for relatively low wages. The crash and resulting economic turmoil took a significant toll. Patient census declined precipitously. By 1933, one survey showed nearly half of the beds in nonprofit hospitals were empty.

Meanwhile, public hospitals like Grady were being kept busy, with occupancy rates that same year approaching 90 percent. Between 1929 and 1933, municipal hospitals saw a patient population increase of 21 percent. It would have been good news, except that the increase seemed to be primarily driven by nonpaying patients. The increase in local government funding in no way matched the increased patient load.

The very existence of prepaid hospital insurance altered forever the uneasy relationship between nonprofit hospitals and their public, government-owned counterparts. The nonprofits could now determine what level of free care to the poor and uninsured they could afford. It was based, at least in part, by how much money they could make on the deals they cut with insurance plans and their covered patients.

Public hospitals were free to try to cut the same deals. But they had no such prerogative when it came to the poor and uninsured. They had to treat whoever showed up. They were the designated safety net for American medicine.

More Hospitals in More Places

Born in Central Georgia in 1882, James Griffin Boswell lived through the economic turmoil of Reconstruction in the South, through the New Deal era, and beyond World War II. He founded the J. G. Boswell Co., which once was the nation's largest cotton producer.

Boswell was the son of a Georgia legislator. He also was a colonel in the US Army, who lived long enough to see his native Greene County, Georgia—and the counties around it— go from a wealthy, plantation economy run by whites to an impoverished, economically dependent community where two of every three residents were black.

He eventually left Georgia for California, where he was a generous benefactor to the California Institute of Technology and other colleges. But before he died in 1952, he had a longtime philanthropic goal yet to achieve. He wanted a hospital to be built back home in Georgia and named for his mother, Minnie.

Getting local government leaders to help foot the bill was all but impossible. Greene County was tiny, with a population of only about 16,000 people. Neighboring counties were even smaller, and poorer. They could barely afford public schools, let alone a hospital.

But Boswell kept pushing, using his connections at the Georgia capital in Atlanta and his personal fortune to help finance the project. As World War II ended and President Harry Truman pressed Congress to take dramatic action and enact a national health insurance plan, based on the success achieved by Social Security, Boswell and Georgia's political leadership saw an opening.

The debate over national health insurance, like those around the time of World War I and at the dawn of the New Deal, took on now very familiar talking points. And, as it had twice before, Truman's progressive idea—he argued it was not only a moral, but also an economic imperative—formulated into legislation nonetheless got buried in opposition.

Compulsory health insurance wasn't needed. It was socialistic in nature, and the country had just fought a war against the tyranny of a national dictatorship that had ruined Germany. The doctors were against it. The hospitals were against it. The growing commercial insurance industry was really against it. Even the unions, which had grown accustomed to negotiating health insurance benefits in lieu of suppressed wages, were against it.

But to provide Truman something of a victory, his Democratic colleagues in the US Senate agreed to one of his other legislative initiatives: rebuilding aging hospitals that had suffered from lack of funding during the war and stimulating the growth of hospitals in rural areas where there were none.

Senator Lister Hill of Alabama became a major promoter of the plan. The son of an Alabama surgeon who studied under famed microbiologist Joseph Lister (hence the senator's first name), Hill had spoken often and eloquently on the Senate floor about how nearly half of the nation's counties lacked hospital facilities. He had bipartisan backing from Senator Harold Burton, a Republican from Ohio who cosponsored the legislation.

Their bill to provide federal funding for hospital construction was going nowhere until Truman weighed in with his plan for national health insurance.

It was then that the American Hospital Association, an ardent opponent of Truman's health insurance plan, enlisted Burton's Ohio colleague, Senator Howard Taft, to push the hospital construction bill as an alternative.

Taft drew up a funding formula for construction funds to be based on population and per capita income with the most needy counties to be served first. That meant that the South's counties would likely have the best chance for getting the federal largesse, significantly weakening any opposition.

When legislators from the North and the large cities of the South objected that the bill ignored the needs of poor patients being served by hospitals in their areas, Hill and Burton inserted language into the measure requiring a "reasonable" amount of free or reduced charges (the bill did not define *reasonable*) for poor patients in any hospital that received federal funds. Largely by default, the federal government was about to establish the first real provision—as weak as it was—into law requiring most hospitals to provide some level of free care.

Despite being heavily weighted toward Southern counties, Hill had to do one other thing to secure the votes of fellow Democrats from his region. He added a provision that permitted hospitals receiving the money to segregate patients by race—justifying it on the basis that the facilities for blacks may be separate, but should be equal to what was available for whites. (This one provision of the Hill–Burton Act marked the first time in the twentieth century that racial segregation was codified in federal law. It would come into play in a big way a few years later when the Grady Memorial Hospital that exists today was built with two separate wings for whites and blacks. The segregation provision of the act stayed on the books until 1963 when it was struck down by federal courts.)

Georgia Gets in Line for Rural Hospital Help

The first round of funding for the Hill–Burton Act would be for five years at $75 million a year in federal funds provided to local governments that applied for it and could prove they had the ability to pay their portion of construction, as well as a plan to keep the hospital solvent.

The state of Georgia jumped in quickly, approving plans for hospitals in eight different locations, the smallest of which was Greene County.

In February of 1948, the US Surgeon General—then in charge of the program—approved construction funds for a twenty-eight-bed hospital in Greensboro, Georgia. Under the funding formula approved by Congress, the Hill–Burton Act paid $133,750 for the hospital. Neither the state nor Greene County could afford to make the match needed to get the hospital started. But J. G. Boswell could. He covered the remaining cost of construction, doubling the amount put up by the Feds. A little over a year later the $400,000 Minnie G. Boswell Memorial Hospital was dedicated in Greensboro.

The same year the Greensboro hospital got the money, four other hospitals on Georgia's list were approved. The following year, the other three Georgia hospitals got their funding. The state, which a decade earlier had turned its back on much of

FDR's New Deal funding for employment and health programs, seemed comfortable now with the federal government subsidizing hospital construction.

In the first fifteen years of the Hill–Burton Act, Georgia, Mississippi, and Arkansas led the South and indeed the nation in new hospital construction, thanks to the law. This was federal money state leaders were more than happy to accept.

By 1975, expenditures under the Hill–Burton Act no longer were needed. The private capital market was more open to health care investment by then, especially among well-established nonprofits. Still, in the time it was up and running, the act had helped finance 9,200 new medical facilities (nursing homes, rehab centers, even outpatient departments were added in 1954) with a total of 416,000 beds.

In hindsight, the frenzy toward rural hospital construction that Hill–Burton started probably had some unintended consequences. Local governments, especially after the enactment of Medicare in the 1960s, began to see hospitals as an economic development investment. In rural communities, having a doctor or two practicing in town was not enough. The doctor would need a place to admit his Medicare patients when they needed minor surgery or intravenous drips to administer drugs and fluids. Without one, the physician would have to send his patients fifty to seventy-five miles away and likely turn over care to another doctor. Without a local hospital, the chances of recruiting doctors to underserved areas were slim. Additionally, hospitals could become an employment base in rural counties without large industries.

By the mid-1970s, many local governments had formed hospital authorities authorized to issue bonds to get their counties in the game. Some of them got matching Hill–Burton money, but most were on their own.

In Hancock County, adjacent to Greene County in Georgia, local officials wanted their own hospital. In 1968 they raised the funds to build a fifty-bed facility to be used by the two private physicians in the county seat of Sparta and open, as well, to the low-income patients who got their care at a federally funded public health clinic in town.

Six years later, it was in deep trouble. The Medicare patients it was admitting did not nearly cover its cost of operations. It took in some Medicaid patients, but the reimbursement it got from the state's Medicaid program was woeful. Interestingly, many of the uninsured patients who were being seen at the federal health clinic were choosing to go to Augusta, which was fifty miles away, when they needed hospitalization. In Augusta, the public hospital would not send them a bill.

In 1974 Hancock Memorial closed down. But it wasn't dead yet. The county hired a Tennessee company to reopen it and take over operations. Still, the average daily census was dismal. On any given night, there would be fewer than ten patients getting care.

It shouldn't have been a surprise. Hancock County was exceedingly poor, with every new census study showing it was either the most impoverished or second most impoverished county in Georgia. It had fewer than a hundred businesses, employing fewer than one thousand workers. (Most of the population worked outside the county.)

There were efforts to change the hospital's operating license with the state to convert some of the beds from acute care to nursing care, a "swing bed" plan that would allow the administration to increase or reduce staffing based on demand.

It limped along for about fifteen years with the same business model. Hospital authority officials and the Hancock County Commission sought other companies to run it, but by 2000 the debt was piling up to the point it was insolvent. A new company devised a plan to close it temporarily and get the state to change the hospital's operating license once again, this time designating it a critical access facility. That would reduce the number of beds from fifty to fifteen.

But that didn't work either. The hospital was underwater

from bad debt, legal judgments against it, and overpayment for tens of thousands of dollars from Medicare that the federal agency said went for unnecessary care.

In March 2001, it closed its doors again, promising to reopen in ninety days. It's still closed.

Remarkably, local officials until recently were still holding out hope that they could sell the building to a larger health care system in a nearby town that might want a satellite. This is what the Minnie G. Boswell Memorial Hospital did in neighboring Greene County, when in 2004 it sold the first Hill–Burton hospital to a Miami, Florida, company, which in turn sold it in 2008 to St. Joseph's Hospital in Atlanta, which merged with Emory Healthcare in 2011. Emory, in turn, sold it to St. Mary's Health Care, an Athens nonprofit health system.

Hancock Memorial was one of the first rural hospitals in Georgia to shutter its doors in the new millennium. It would not be the last.

5

RACE, MEDICARE, AND MEDICAID

In the early 1960s, Grady Memorial Hospital was one of the most visible symbols of the nation's separate-but-equal approach to race relations. Although that status may have been quietly accepted in Atlanta at the time, it would not survive for long.

The painful march toward civil rights, a movement that was birthed in Atlanta, was well under way. In the middle of the tumultuous decade, the federal government would intervene and use its considerable power to fundamentally alter public policy regarding race in both the public accommodations and health care arenas. Ultimately, the health provisions of these legislative changes would fall short of the goal of securing medical care for poor blacks, as well as poor whites. But they nonetheless changed how hospitals were run.

In 1958, a new $20-million, sixteen-story hospital opened to replace the rundown White Grady and Black Grady buildings on either side of Butler Street in the heart of Atlanta. Viewed from the sky, the modern hospital resembled a giant three-dimensional *H*, with patient rooms on both sides and a connecting corridor with banks of elevators between them.

The hospital was bustling with patients. Nearly eight thousand babies were delivered there in 1958, making it one of the largest obstetrics hospitals in the country. Most of the beds in other wards were filled too, pretty evenly occupied between blacks and whites. There were seventeen surgical suites handling trauma and routine operations. The nursing staff—half white, half black (whose student nurses lived in new, segregated dorms nearby)—was busy caring for patients of their own color, each in their respective sides of the building.

Shuttling between the two wings were about five hundred teaching physicians, residents, medical students, and visiting doctors—all of them white. They served in a Noah's Ark–type hospital with at least two of everything—radiology departments, laboratories, blood banks, operating rooms, emergency units—all set up that way solely for the purpose of keeping black patients separated from white patients.

Services in the hospital chapel were strictly separated. The hospital's chaplain was white, and he was instructed not to integrate services. If black families wanted a clergyman to say a prayer in the chapel with them, they could call on a black preacher.

Still, there were some day-to-day logistics that the modern design of the new Grady failed to take into account. Laundry handling was one of them.

Laundry chutes for the tall building were located in the connecting corridors. It just wouldn't be right, administrators decided, to mix the soiled bed linens from black and white patients down the same chutes. Their plan: Alternate the days when linens from the white patients and those from the black patients would be sent down the chute to the basement laundry. (Ironically, once it got there, all the laundry work in the hospital was done by black women.)

Grady Memorial Hospital may have finally gotten the new, modern facility it wanted—and Atlanta needed—but it was still, as the city's residents had grown accustomed to calling it, "The Gradys."

Desegregating the Gradys

But by the end of the decade, Henry W. Grady Memorial Hospital would rid itself of these and many other artifacts of the Jim Crow era. It did so in a typically Atlanta way, with behind-the-scenes negotiating between black and white leaders, combined with steady and effective confrontation by activists who never let their activism turn violent.

Here's how it unfolded.

At the beginning of the 1960s, the city had roughly three thousand acute-care beds in more than a dozen hospitals. Most of those facilities were restricted—some purposely, most informally—to white patients. It wasn't necessarily explicit racism at work, so much as it was the inevitable consequence of hospital rules that required a physician to admit patients. And the reality was that Atlanta's predominantly white physician force saw very few black patients.

Instead, most black patients, disproportionately poor and uninsured, had made Grady their medical home, because many of them gained admission to the hospital when they showed up in distress at the emergency room doors. Civil rights historians still debate whether this result was by default or by design. But it was a fact. And this bitter history influences the politics of support for public hospitals to this day, especially in the South, where similar scenarios played out during this same time.

While enrollment of black students in major medical schools was beginning to expand in other parts of the country, it was not in much of the South. Atlanta's handful of black doctors at the time were educated in all-black medical schools in other parts of the country. When they set up practice in Atlanta, they tended to admit their patients to three tiny, all-black hospitals in the city, none of which was accredited for care by independent or government agencies.

By this time as well, Grady had been transferred from control by the city to a hospital authority appointed by the county commissioners from Fulton and DeKalb counties, who were responsible for subsidizing the cost of caring for the poor.

Grady's advocates had hoped that an independent authority would remove the hospital from city politics, which, they were convinced, contributed to the hospital's chronic inability to persuade Atlanta voters to pay for bond issues to improve the hospital. (The change proved initially to be true, but it didn't insulate the hospital for long. Over the years, the new governance structure created a new round of political dramas that would jeopardize Grady's future.) Still, the new authority had the state's permission to issue bonds without voter approval. There seems little question that without the change, the new hospital might never have been built.

Like other cities around the country, the Atlanta metro area was discovering its suburbs. New highways, spurred by the availability of federal funds through the Interstate Highway Act in the 1950s, connected small towns in the ring around Atlanta via a hub-and-spokes network that made it easier for people to live outside the city but work inside it.

Surrounding counties had established hospitals to serve their growing populations, which were overwhelmingly white, while Atlanta's population was well on its way toward becoming majority black. Most significantly, several of Atlanta's established hospitals—among them, St. Joseph's, the city's first—were considering moving to new locations outside the city.

Moreover, Emory University's medical school had ambitions of its own and wasn't exactly sure where Grady—its primary teaching hospital—fit into its long-range plans.

By the 1960s, Emory was the only medical school in the city. It was building a reputation in medical science as well as clinical care. Emory operated Emory University Hospital on its academic campus in suburban Atlanta. That hospital was built in 1922 (when it was known as Wesley Memorial Hospital) on the strength of a $1.25 million gift from Coca-Cola founder (and Emory trustee) Asa Candler.

Additionally, Emory had acquired a nonprofit hospital named after Crawford W. Long (the Georgian who is credited with the first use of surgical anesthesia), which was less than two miles from Grady in downtown Atlanta. Emory physicians had admission privileges at both hospitals.

Grady, with its diverse pool of patients, served as the perfect learning environment for medical students and residents, and Emory had no intention of abandoning it. Indeed, the school and the hospital authority signed the first long-term contract for Emory's exclusive medical staff services in 1951. But a decade later, the epicenter of hospital care and public health moved closer to the Emory campus.

In the years before World War II, the federal government began to turn its attention to prevention of easily spread diseases that military personnel faced while serving overseas—and sometimes at home. One of these was malaria, which showed up from time to time in outbreaks around military installations in the South. Coastal Georgia and other swampy Southern regions were breeding grounds for epidemics. The federal government, going back to the New Deal era, had established laboratories and dispatched experts to help the states deal with them.

The CDC Is Formed

After the war, the effort was greatly expanded. The US Surgeon General and the national Public Health Service were put in charge of a new agency, the Communicable Disease Center, which needed a home. Robert W. Woodruff, who purchased the Coca-Cola company from the Candler family and was himself a great benefactor of Emory University, had just the place. Woodruff worked behind the scenes to get Emory to donate fifteen acres on the north end of its Druid Hills campus to the federal government for the new agency's home base.

Woodruff had a keen interest in malaria. He owned a plantation in south Georgia, Ichauway, in an area where farmhands and tenant farmers routinely came in contact with the disease. The wealthy business executive was intent on keeping malaria in check by, among other ways, making quinine readily available to everyone in Baker County. He also provided funds to the Emory medical school to study malaria and its Georgia victims.

Still, it was more than a decade before the Public Health Service broke ground on the heavily wooded area Woodruff had in mind to construct the first laboratories and administrative offices for what eventually became the Centers for Disease Control and Prevention (CDC). The proximity to campus of a new federal health agency devoted to identifying and controlling infectious diseases and studying patterns in the cause of chronic disease, and the growth of Emory University Hospital, transformed the area surrounding the university's Clifton Road location into one of the nation's largest specialty care and medical research corridors.

The disease-tracking experts at the CDC could share joint appointments with the new agency and the medical school. Faculty physicians and researchers affiliated with the medical school on Clifton Road had offices near the University Hospital. In 1990, Emory opened a school of public health, only a block away from the CDC on Clifton Road, supporting many research and teaching affiliations.

Indeed, in 2014 the connection between Emory and the CDC captured worldwide attention when the first two American medical volunteers from Ebola-stricken West Africa were flown to Atlanta to be treated for the disease in a specially prepared room at Emory University Hospital.

Medical schools around the country were making similar moves during this time. Although the schools were still affiliated with public hospitals for teaching purposes, the pace of new drug development, new surgical procedures, and other advances in clinical care was accelerating so fast it was difficult for faculty members to divide their time among teaching, practicing, and doing research.

At their own hospitals, the medical schools' administrators would be fully in charge and their faculty not subject to the whims and political influence of administrators appointed by public officials. New surgical procedures that attracted great attention from the media, such as open-heart surgery and organ transplantation, could be studied and performed at the university hospitals, greatly enhancing the medical schools' reputations.

Moreover, as access and affordability of health insurance began to grow among middle-class Americans, these highly sought patients would not have to share hospital space with the poor and uninsured in the public teaching hospitals. The medical schools could easily create teaching programs in their own hospitals, if they so desired.

In cities around the country, these decisions altered the relationship between the medical schools and many public hospitals in ways it would take some years to fully comprehend. But the bottom line was that university hospitals became competitors with the public hospitals their faculty and students staffed. In many cities where public hospitals struggle to get paying patients today, this remains the case.

With Emory's medical school faculty being all white and most of the private hospitals admitting mostly white, insured patients, the stage was set for a confrontation about what was happening at Grady in the early 1960s.

Black activists, especially the students at Atlanta's black colleges, had heard too many stories about extremely ill patients being sent home from the emergency room because there were no more black beds available while dozens of white beds were empty.

Negro Ambulances

There was a report in a black newspaper about a boy hit by a car near Morehouse College (Martin Luther King Jr.'s alma mater) who lay injured in the street because Grady said there were no "Negro ambulances" available to come get him. They knew Grady workers were required to use a "colored laborer's cafeteria" for meals. (Indeed, there were segregated meal rooms for black nurses and black nursing students at Grady. But there was also a second tier of segregation between the medical help and all other black employees—maids, porters, even the very workers who staffed the kitchens.) Moreover, another black newspaper reported these same workers were earning hourly wages that were half of what white workers were paid.

The black students in the city arranged a meeting with the hospital's administrators. When they got there, they found the Reverend Martin Luther King—"Daddy King," as he was known—who urged them to back off their protests against the hospital and give the administrators time to make changes.

The students remained distrustful. After all, Frank Wilson, Grady's chief administrator—a former city council member who had helped the hospital achieve some national recognition for its services—had reportedly proclaimed that he would "die and go to hell" before Grady was integrated.

In June of 1962, the local chapter of the NAACP sued Grady to desegregate. Among the plaintiffs was a black physician who wanted admitting privileges at the hospital, a Spelman College student who said she wanted to attend a desegregated nursing school, and several city residents who said as potential patients they were entitled to the same level of care, in the same facilities, as white patients.

The case was fought over the separate-but-equal concept (although that language was rarely used in court or depositions), with Grady's lawyers claiming black patients were getting the same care as whites. The phrase most often used to describe the arrangement was "nondiscriminatory but separate." Wilson argued in a deposition, for instance, that ambulance dispatchers needed to know the race of the potential patient because some of the private ambulance services the hospital used didn't accept black patients. Regardless, Wilson flatly declared in his deposition that separation of the patients by race was "in the best interest of the physical, mental health, and well-being of all patients."

It wasn't a compelling defense, and Atlanta's power structure—led by the business community and assisted by respected black leaders—saw it was a losing one, especially in light of what was happening in Washington with the passage of the Civil Rights Act in 1964. They prevailed on Wilson and other Grady leaders to begin to make changes.

The emergency department was the first to desegregate. A handful of black physicians received "visiting staff" privileges at Grady. The first black intern came on board. "Black" and "White" signs on doors to laboratories and emergency rooms disappeared. The hospital got its first black chaplain. Black and white nurses wore the same uniforms.

But the lawsuit remained active during all this. Under pressure from a federal judge, the nursing programs were integrated and other separate-but-equal programs at the hospital went quietly away. Administrators were most worried about the last phase of integration—moving black and white patients around the hospital to share rooms. But it went off without a struggle.

Interestingly, that happened only a few months after Frank Wilson—the man who had declared he would be dead and in hell before Grady integrated—died of a heart attack.

Remnants of Grady's segregated past lingered for years, but the battle had been largely won.

By the 1980s, Emory's medical staff at the hospital was joined by the staff of a new medical school, the Morehouse School of Medicine, chartered as an institution dedicated to producing physicians to practice in minority and underserved communities. It was something of a shotgun marriage arranged by a growing and powerful group of black elected leaders in Atlanta, Emory, and Grady, which was then still controlled by a mostly white hospital authority board.

The two medical schools couldn't have been more different. Emory argued that Morehouse—because of its size and charter—would not be able to adequately staff some of the hospital's more intensive services. But the three partners eventually cut a deal for Morehouse faculty and students to use Grady as a teaching facility, helping to staff its internal medicine and other primary care services and work toward eventually getting placements in the more specialized departments.

The Grady deal helped solidify Morehouse's future. Morehouse School of Medicine leaders went on to become high-ranking federal health officials, including former MMS presidents Dr. Louis Sullivan, who was health and human services secretary under President George H. W. Bush, and US Surgeon General Dr. David Satcher, who served under President Bill Clinton.

Still, it would take forces well outside of Atlanta to force the full integration of the city's other hospitals after Grady broke the barriers in 1963. The Civil Rights Act of 1964 played a big role, but the federal law that came next sealed the deal.

Medicare, Medicaid, and the Half-Baked Cake

The same year Grady was integrated marked a major change in the role played by the federal government—and to a much-less-well-understood role, by the states—in America's unfinished business of guaranteeing everyone access to health care.

The story of how President Lyndon B. Johnson pushed his ambitious plan for Medicare through Congress is well known to most Americans, especially the baby boomers who are now coming to enjoy its benefits. But what is less known is how Medicare altered the government's relationship with America's hospitals—creating a financial footing that secured healthy operating margins for most of them, but at the same time making them play by Washington's rules.

Among other requirements, the federal government codified a very simple policy for hospitals: In order to receive

Medicare dollars, blacks and whites must be treated equally and in the same—not separate—facilities.

If there was any significant resistance among hospitals to this strong-arming by the Feds, it evaporated fairly quickly. The prospect of guaranteed payment for all elderly Americans—about half of them at the time were not covered by insurance—was too enticing, even for hospitals that only a few years earlier strictly prohibited the admission of blacks. For others like Grady with separate facilities, the new rule made it easier to persuade reluctant administrators to accept full integration.

Little wonder. The landmark Medicare law amounted to the first time that the nation's political leadership, in the form of the President of the United States and Congress, acknowledged the need to guarantee at least one segment of the American population access to health care.

Written as an amendment to the Social Security Act, the new law created a financing plan, with taxes levied and managed by the federal government, to pay for a huge new social program. Besides a monthly pension, with the enactment of Medicare, the government now assured Americans over the age of sixty-five that nearly all their hospital bills would be covered when they needed care.

Moreover, there was nothing "voluntary" about this government program. With few exceptions, every elderly American would be covered, and every American worker's paycheck would get a chunk taken out of it to pay for the plan. The concept of "compulsory" health insurance—the unrealized goal of progressives in the country going back to World War I—was now in place, even if most of the workers compelled to pay for it would not qualify for it for years to come. Like their parents had with Social Security three decades earlier, a new generation of Americans was now paying for a new social program for their elders.

While the American Medical Association and well-known conservatives such as Ronald Reagan were enlisted to fight

Medicare, the nation's hospitals and their trade organizations embraced the prospect. Who could blame them? The legislation was written in a way that guaranteed that all "reasonable costs" would be included in the reimbursement rates for hospital services to Medicare beneficiaries.

Indeed, the financing arm for the program, the Medicare Trust Fund, was limited to payments for hospital services. If elderly Americans wanted insurance to cover physician services, they could pay premiums through their Social Security checks for Medicare Part B, but that coverage was strictly voluntary. (Initially, very few did, even though their premium costs were subsidized by general revenue from federal taxes. Part B had deductibles, and there was no limit on out-of-pocket costs for physician services.)

But acceptance of Part A, coverage of hospitalization, was nearly universal. The program paid for up to ninety days of hospital care per illness and up to one hundred days of skilled nursing home care for extended services, if needed for recovery. (This last provision sparked a boom in the nursing home industry that was even bigger than the boost Medicare provided to hospitals. Some of the new, for-profit nursing home companies—Humana, Inc., being among the most well known—eventually morphed into highly profitable hospital chains, thanks in large part to the assurances of Medicare reimbursement.)

With nearly half of all adult Americans now covered by insurance they purchased through their workplace, and the vast majority of elders covered by Medicare, hospitals had achieved the footing they needed to increase size, hire more nurses and staff, and purchase the latest technology.

With the assurance of Medicare and the help of hospital authorities—quasi-governmental agencies that could tap the bond market for capital—affluent suburban counties could finance their own hospitals without providing operating subsidies like those needed by the less-affluent urban counties for their public hospitals. Indeed, federal money from the Hill–Burton Act for hospital construction was still flowing. And the states, which played a major role in deciding who got Hill–Burton funds, threw money toward suburban hospital construction the way they used federal dollars to help build new highways in growing metro areas.

In the twenty-year span between 1950 and 1970—only four years after Medicare was implemented—hospital employment in the United States more than doubled.

While Medicare may have been the largest publicly financed health care plan to date, it still had uniquely American characteristics owing to the nation's long-standing deference to local control. Federal law stipulated the benefit plan and costs. But Washington allowed local communities to decide how to "administer" the day-to-day logistics of filing claims and paying benefits.

Not looking to create new bureaucracies, the states were encouraged—indeed pushed by the hospitals that would benefit most—to let local hospitals choose Blue Cross and Blue Shield associations to administer Medicare claims. The Blues, which the nonprofit hospital industry helped create, would be a much better administrator of the new program than Prudential, or Metropolitan Life, or one of the for-profit commercial insurers, the hospitals argued. Whatever operating surplus they achieved by administering the plans could be reinvested into future plans to keep costs low.

This logic prevailed. And with Medicare plans in their portfolio of products, the Blue Cross and Blue Shield associations around the country became the dominant force in health insurance.

A Government Plan Takes Hold

Medicare was an unquestionable success at achieving its goal of securing health care access for the nation's oldest citizens. There is great debate over how much of a role it played in increasing the life-span of Americans after it was implemented, but there seems little question it had a positive impact. Life expectancy in the United States and elsewhere in the industrialized world had begun to markedly improve, thanks to advances in medicine and public health. But with health insurance now readily available to some of the country's most vulnerable citizens, the average life-span of Americans increased by fifteen years between 1965 and 1984.

Moreover, the landmark legislation signed by President Johnson in 1965 had taken into account nearly all the goals the progressive reformers fifty years earlier had been advocating to make the United States more like European nations in assuring their citizens of the health and welfare they need when they need it.

The United States now had compulsory unemployment insurance and government-backed Social Security to provide a pension for the elderly. Medicare was described as a "three-layer cake" that was supposed to complete the mission.

Parts A and B were in place to cover hospital and physician bills for the elderly, and the third layer, Medicaid (they never called it Part C, for some reason), was going to deal with the one population—the poor—that had always represented the biggest stumbling block toward a true national health plan.

Why this three-layer cake crumbled remains the subject of great debate that nearly always breaks down by whether you think it was a good idea in the first place. But it is also a uniquely American story of political partisanship, unintended consequences, marketplace maneuvering, and the still widely held belief that government involvement in health care should be limited as much as possible.

Medicaid as Welfare

The key turning point in this story is Medicaid, which is why it's important to go back a few years before it was enacted.

Medicare for the elderly was a concept that had gained widespread acceptance in opinion polls during the presidential campaign in 1960. Indeed, the young Democratic candidate, John F. Kennedy, talked often about it. But opponents in Congress, the AMA, and others who continued to believe the market and public charity would better serve the country than a public program saw the trend line of public option and took a big step to defuse it that year.

The House Ways and Means Committee Chairman, Wilbur Mills of Ohio, and his counterpart in the Senate, Robert Kerr of Oklahoma, drafted legislation to extend the small federal subsidies Washington was giving the states to use for welfare programs aimed at covering some of the medical bills for the poor and elderly.

The Kerr–Mills Act, which swept through Congress, provided between 50 to 80 percent of the funds the states would need to subsidize health care to the elderly poor if the states decided they wanted to participate. Moreover, the states would also get to create the "means test"—the metric used to determine if someone was truly worthy—to be eligible for the funds.

Predictably, the states balked at signing up for the act. Only five large states accounted for 90 percent of the Kerr–Mills spending in the first three years. Most of the other states were not interested in creating a new yearly budget item to match the Kerr–Mills money they were getting from Washington.

Besides, they said, who knew whether Washington would stay true to its promise of funds? Once the elderly poor had gotten used to health care coverage, they would not want to give it up, leaving the states to pay the full freight, they argued. (If this argument sounds familiar, it's because it is the same talking point Obamacare opponents raise today regarding expansion of Medicaid, despite the fact the law requires the federal government to pay no less than 90 percent of expansion costs in the first ten years of its existence.)

Kerr–Mills had its intended effect, however, since it was really a tactic to delay the rush toward Medicare. But the year after Kennedy's death with Johnson at the peak of his power, the same opponents saw they did not have enough votes to stop its enactment. Instead, they promoted a Kerr–Mills–like plan as the basis for the third layer of the cake. LBJ and his allies cut a deal. While the federal government would provide the bulk of the money for Medicaid—a new program that covered poor Americans, including infants, children, and their very poor parents—the states would run it and decide who would qualify.

The language employed at the time to describe Americans qualifying for both programs was descriptive of the ideology behind them. You can still hear these same labels today. Medicare has "beneficiaries." Medicaid has "recipients." One group had earned its privilege of health care coverage. The other group was not so worthy. Indeed, if they are to receive the government's help, it should only be temporary.

Fifty years later, it sounds harsher than it probably did then.

That's why it's worth remembering that throughout its history, this country has always thought that local people, institutions, and public officials are in the best position to determine who needs "poor relief" and who doesn't. It's also why Medicaid should be viewed as a welfare program as much as a medical program, albeit a very costly extension in the way welfare has been administered. By definition, poor relief should be temporary for able-bodied Americans, according to our political and social ethic. By granting any form of guaranteed health care coverage for the nonelderly poor, America would run the risk of making them dependent on the welfare state.

So the theory went then. And so it goes—with a few exceptions—today, especially in the South, where spending on federal programs like unemployment pay, school lunches, food stamps, and Medicaid is always weighed against the risk of creating a dependent class of citizens that will bankrupt the states.

Predictably, giving the states control over Medicaid created a checkerboard pattern of eligibility around the country, as the states—one by one, some of them very reluctantly—signed on to the program. (Arizona didn't join it until 1982.) The law required the states to have a baseline that would cover the poorest of the poor, as well as most infants in low-income families and the disabled of all ages who needed nursing home care. Most states opted not to allow enrollment of those working in low-wage jobs who were not covered by employee plans, nor those who were self-employed.

The decision to cover nursing home costs with Medicaid and not Medicare also altered the trajectory of the program in a way that has had lasting repercussions.

Since Medicare was designed and funded originally as protection from the high cost of hospitalization for the elderly, there was no provision within it stipulating how to pay for long-term care. Medicare does cover a short-term nursing home stay for patients well enough to leave the hospital but still in need of skilled nursing care. But, as the adult children of elderly Americans find out every day, Medicare is not the government program to help them or their parents pay the thousands of dollars per month it takes to pay for nursing home care.

Not long after Medicare was enacted, it became obvious that many of the elderly—especially those very old Americans who could not care for themselves at home—would need institutional care, many of them for the rest of their lives. Similarly, Congress agreed that a government program should cover those who were permanently disabled and unable to work, regardless of age.

They decided that program was Medicaid.

In theory, turning to Medicaid seemed logical even if, as

a practical matter, implementing it seemed especially harsh on many families. After "spending down" most of their disposable income, the new regulations said, elderly and disabled people needing nursing home care could qualify as poor enough to get Medicaid. Indeed, Medicaid funds could be used to pay their Medicare premiums and other out-of-pocket expenses not covered by Medicare.

But over the years, the cost of paying for nursing home care under Medicaid has come to heavily weigh against the program designed originally as a health insurance plan for the poor. Indeed there are now nearly ten million "dual eligible" enrollees in Medicaid—those elderly and disabled whose hospital bills are paid for by Medicare, but whose nursing home services are paid by Medicaid. The services they need represent nearly 40 percent of all Medicaid spending. Medicaid now covers about one in every five Medicare enrollees.

Moreover, several studies have shown that only five percent of enrollees in Medicaid account for nearly half (47 percent) of all Medicaid expenditures. The high individual cost of these patients is driven by their need for acute care, long-term care, or both.

Including long-term care for the elderly in Medicaid—rather than creating a separate program for it, or financing it through Medicare—has been a huge contributor to the escalating cost of state Medicaid budgets.

Lowballing Medicaid Reimbursement

To keep their portion of Medicaid's costs somewhat in check, the states have basically one option, controlling how much they pay hospitals, physicians, and nursing homes that treat Medicaid patients.

Predictably, again in states that never were happy with the program in the first place, the Medicaid rates were set artificially low—much lower than what hospitals and doctors were getting for taking care of Medicare patients and those covered by group health plans. The law made it difficult for hospitals to reject Medicaid patients who came through their doors; they could risk their Medicare reimbursement if they did. So some hospitals devised ways to screen out Medicaid patients before admission.

Bowing to the AMA and other doctor groups, there was no similar incentive in the law for physicians to take Medicaid patients. And when the states lowballed them in reimbursement schedules, many doctors simply chose not to participate.

To some degree, the legislation attempted to make provisions for this. Part of the law was designed to expand a network of federally sponsored community health centers where there were high concentrations of poor and uninsured people. Most of these were in rural areas. Some opened in poorer sections of cities as well. The effort was ultimately hampered when Congress did not appropriate enough money to make many of them viable.

The centers were to be staffed by young physicians paying off medical school loans, and they were required by the law to take Medicaid patients. But because of chronic shortfalls in their operating budgets, they also relied on getting a healthy dose of Medicare and privately insured patients. Medicaid alone could not sustain them.

This third layer of the health-care-for-all cake—with its mushy batter mixed up and sloppily layered onto Medicare by the states—caused the whole cake to tilt. And the mess it created wound up in the laps of the nation's public hospitals.

With private-practice doctors turning Medicaid patients away, they went to the one place they knew would treat them even for basic health needs—the emergency room of the public hospital. Moreover, with Medicare now covering nearly all the elderly, these patients—including the aged poor—had a real choice of hospitals for care. They were no longer dependent on the public hospital. When they moved to private, nonprofit hospitals, they took their Medicare cards with them. In one of the many ironies of health policy decision-making, Medicare's enactment—which many progressives thought would solidify funding for public hospitals—instead put them at a competitive disadvantage with their neighboring private hospitals.

The private hospitals were already dominating the market of commercially insured patients covered through group health plans. Now they were getting a whole new market of elderly patients for whom the federal government had promised to cover all reasonable costs.

Public hospitals got Medicare patients too, but not nearly as many as their private counterparts. The good news for public hospitals was that some of the poor patients they had been treating for free would now have their care paid by Medicaid. The bad news was that the Medicaid rates the states paid for those patients were purposely low, leaving the hospitals still losing money on them. And the worst news was that one other sizable segment of the American population—those able-bodied adults not covered on the job who made too much money to be eligible for Medicaid, but not enough to afford any other health insurance—was left out altogether. Large public hospitals like Grady would remain the safety net to catch them when they were sick.

Once again, these institutions were left serving the half-baked cake that has come to represent the unfinished business of American health care reform.

6
GETTING TO NOW

If you were a universal health insurance advocate and blinked in the early 1970s, you may have missed it. For one brief moment, there was a bipartisan effort to fill in the coverage gaps left after the enactment of Medicare and Medicaid.

It involved President Richard Nixon, the conservative Republican who had already stunned his supporters in his first term by opening up diplomatic relations with China. This time his diplomacy was aimed at the liberal Democratic lion and best-known promoter of national health insurance, Senator Edward M. Kennedy of Massachusetts.

As he neared reelection in 1972, Nixon suggested that American employers be required to provide insurance coverage for their workers. That was heresy enough to many Republicans at the time, but Nixon went a big step further, calling for a public program for everyone not covered by Medicare, Medicaid, or job-related insurance. By February of 1974, Nixon was calling comprehensive health insurance "an idea whose time has come."

Deep in the throes of the Watergate scandal, Richard Nixon was clearly searching for a domestic legacy achievement. He and his aides spent more than a year reaching out to Kennedy, who had a plan of his own. It was similar to Medicare in concept—financed with federal taxes—but it would have been open to anyone who wanted to purchase it. Kennedy, assisted by the powerful chairman of the House Ways and Means Committee, Wilbur Mills, began serious negotiations with the Nixon White House to come up with a bipartisan plan.

Despite misgivings by liberal supporters about Nixon's intentions, Kennedy said in June of 1974 that there was a "new spirit of compromise in the air."

But yet another round of revelations about Watergate and illegal activities covered up by Nixon and his aides crippled the White House a few weeks later. All negotiations on a health care bill came to a halt. Nixon resigned in August of that year.

It was over almost before it began, yet another failure to move the United States into the growing class of wealthy and industrial nations that have some form of universal health care for its citizens.

Nixon's failure ushered in a new era of incrementalism in health care reform that was to last nearly two decades. No one—save Kennedy—promoted comprehensive reform in any meaningful way during this time.

The best Congress could muster in the Jimmy Carter, Ronald Reagan, and George H. W. Bush years was a provision that allowed workers who lost jobs where they had been covered by insurance a way to keep it, at full cost, and without the previous employer's contribution. The idea was to tide them over temporarily until they found another job, one hopefully that came with insurance.

But without the employer subsidy, the cost of these plans was exorbitant, and many workers chose to go without. And as manufacturing jobs with good benefits diminished, many of the laid-off workers settled for employment in retail and service jobs, which often did not come with insurance.

Also, during the Reagan–Bush years Congress enacted legislation that was designed to assist hospitals that cared for a "disproportionate share" of the poor and uninsured by providing them a higher level of Medicare reimbursement based on the state's poverty level, the uninsured rate, and the volume of uncompensated care the hospitals provided. This too was considered a stopgap measure, to help some large public hospitals that were clearly struggling to stay afloat. But it became a semipermanent fixture in federal funding and morphed considerably over the years.

That's because, once again, the states had a major role in implementing a federal policy aimed at providing better health care access for the poor. States were allowed to divvy up the pool of DSH (disproportionate share hospital) funds from the federal government largely as they saw fit. And over the years, the "Lake Wobegon" effect has clearly taken place. More than half of the nation's five thousand licensed hospitals are now deemed to be providing above-average levels of uncompensated care and are therefore eligible for DSH funds. In some states, virtually every hospital was above average and getting DSH funds.

By spreading out the payments so widely, hospitals that truly handled a high number of poor and uninsured patients—hospitals like Grady in Atlanta and other large public hospitals that provided expensive services on a charity basis—were clearly shortchanged. And, as badly distributed as these funds are even today, many hospitals are heavily dependent on getting their disproportionate share money. The creation of the disproportionate share program, and the subsequent reliance on it by many hospitals, would play a huge role twenty-five years later in the most recent health reform effort.

"Hillarycare" and the Return of the Socialized Medicine Brand

By the 1990s, with medical costs rising and the number of uninsured Americans steadily climbing, President Bill Clinton came into office vowing to create a comprehensive new plan that would fill in these and other gaping holes in the country's health insurance system. He put First Lady Hillary Clinton, a lawyer by training and an avowed policy wonk, in charge of the effort.

After months of study, the First Lady's plan—created behind the scenes and never fully disclosed—was capsized by yet another wave of "socialized medicine" charges. The same well-funded opponents of compulsory insurance in the past—organized medicine, commercial insurance, and other business interests—quickly dubbed the reform proposals being discussed as "Hillarycare." It wasn't a compliment. By the end of Clinton's first term, the fledgling, comprehensive reform effort had been abandoned.

Instead, opponents of Hillarycare promised that the marketplace would correct most of the problems if insurers were allowed to offer more "affordable" coverage. Affordability, they proclaimed, was the key. If consumers could purchase policies with reasonable premiums, more of them would sign up in the private market. The plans they touted allowed for more managed-care arrangements to control costs, higher deductibles, and out-of-pocket "copayments" so consumers would have more incentive to spend wisely.

Additionally, two new concepts—health savings accounts (HSAs) and high-risk insurance pools—gained some traction among consumers and state regulators.

HSAs allowed workers to set aside an untaxed portion of their paychecks into a fund they could use later to pay medical bills not covered by their insurance. The high-risk pools, set up by the states, were supposedly designed to provide coverage to the chronically ill and otherwise disabled Americans who got turned down for insurance in the private-policy market.

Both concepts got a lot of chatter at state legislatures, where Republicans, in particular, promoted them as alternatives to government regulation of the private insurance market.

Similarly, many state assemblies pushed for tort reform measures on the theory that medical malpractice lawsuits were driving the ever-increasing cost of liability insurance and, by extension, health care costs.

Several states enacted laws limiting the amount juries could award plaintiffs in malpractice cases against physicians. Others made it harder to mount a claim in the first place. Some did both. These reform efforts were supposed to lower the cost of malpractice insurance for physicians, as well as reduce the amount of unnecessary, or "defensive medicine," tests that were driving up the cost of medicine because of fear of litigation.

They helped some, but not much. This should not have been a surprise. A Harvard University study considered by many to be the most authoritative on the issue put the cost of defensive medicine at 2.4 percent of the nation's total health care expenditures. Other studies argue that the cost of medical malpractice insurance accounts for about 1 percent of expenditures.

Nevertheless, the cost of medical care continued significantly to outpace inflation in the economy as a whole during this period. Clearly, these efforts to make insurance more affordable were not working.

Gaming the System

During the Clinton administration and that of George W. Bush, the states got much more creative in devising schemes to maximize federal funding for Medicaid while at the same time trying to minimize the increasing cost of the program to state budgets. Like corporate attorneys looking for loopholes in the tax code, state budget makers poured over the arcane rules for financing Medicaid and found lots of ways to beat the system.

They did this by, among other things, getting hospitals and health care providers to contribute to special trust funds that the state could tap for use as its share of funding for the Medicaid program. These new pools of money allowed the state to demand—and often get—additional federal matching money through the disproportionate share and other federal programs. Most important, they were able to do it without any significant new appropriations from the state treasury.

The result was that many hospitals got back more than what they "contributed" to the state, with little or no direct cost to state taxpayers, which made elected officials quite happy. The hospitals didn't much care for the schemes, but they went along in hopes of reducing their mounting debt for charity care. These Rube Goldberg–like machinations in how money goes into and out of state Medicaid programs would become a standard procedure in the state budget-making process, all aimed at minimizing state expenditures and maximizing the flow of money from Washington to state capitals.

Bill Clinton did accomplish one significant goal during the last years of his presidency: In a deal with a Republican Congress, Clinton arranged for a new program that allowed low-income families to purchase government-subsidized health insurance for children under the age of eighteen.

Unlike Medicaid, where the federal government's portion of the program was based on poverty levels within the state, this time the portion was based on the number of children within the state who were not covered by a family insurance plan. And, also unlike Medicaid, families who signed up for the program could be assessed monthly premiums per child by the states, based on household income.

For their part in managing and paying for the program, states were allowed to determine the maximum income families could make and still qualify and, ultimately, how many children could be enrolled. They also got to set the premium payments.

But almost from the start, the program was financially troubled. The federal government underestimated enrollment, and the projected funding was inadequate. It did not help that some states decided to float income maximums to three to four times above the poverty level—a few even allowed adults to enroll—while others drew the line at two times the poverty level (or about $34,000 a year for a family of four in the year 2000).

By 2007, a decade after it was signed into law, the Children's Health Insurance Program (CHIP) had enrolled 7.2 million people, including 639,000 adults and, in some states, children in families earning $72,000 per year. The federal government's

$5 billion annual contribution was woefully inadequate. The Congressional Budget Office estimated it needed $13.4 billion more that year alone to avoid cutbacks.

Democrats had gained control of the US House of Representatives in the midterm elections of 2006 and were pushing in 2007 for greater funding for the program. Congress passed a reauthorization measure calling for expanding the program to 4 million more children at a cost of $35 billion over the next five years—the increase paid for by a hike in the federal excise tax on cigarettes.

President George W. Bush vetoed the legislation, and the House did not have enough votes to pass it over his objections. The debate turned out to be the precursor to a long line of partisan and ideological disputes that would dominate health care policy discussions in the next administration.

How the states responded to the fiscal challenge posed by CHIP speaks once again to how worthy of help the political leadership in the state believes the working poor to be. It confirms, as well, the uneasy relationship between Washington and the state capitals when it comes to financing social and health programs that are supposed to help the poor.

Lawmakers in some states targeted the program for severe cuts in 2007. In Georgia, the state capped enrollment at 3,000 children per month and required families to have been off private insurance rolls for at least three months before becoming eligible. Georgia's then-speaker of the house proposed clawing back the maximum family income for enrollment to a level that would have been less than two times the poverty line, effectively removing many of the 273,000 children who had signed up. Other states floated similar reduced eligibility plans.

Many states became as disenchanted with CHIP as they were with Medicaid, but they were unable to get rid of it. A new government-subsidized program was in place.

Yet again, the United States had carved out another segment of its population to help gain access to the health care

they needed. Children in low-wage families joined poor pregnant women and their babies, the long-term disabled, and the
elderly as worthy of health coverage backed by the government.
(With a Democrat in the White House and Democrats in control of both houses of Congress, CHIP was reauthorized in
2009 along the lines of the bill that had been vetoed by George
W. Bush two years earlier.)

Still, this patchwork of coverage eligibility for CHIP
matched the results of Medicaid, with some states pulling in
large numbers of uninsured families to get coverage for their
kids, and other states making only a token effort to deal with
the problem.

Similarly, many states elected to control the cost of Medicaid
and CHIP plans by turning to managed-care companies to run
them. Residents on Medicaid and children's health plans were
enrolled in HMO-like plans run by for-profit companies in
contract with the state. Payments to the companies were "cap-
itated," meaning that they were given a flat fee for each person
covered by the state plans. If they managed to keep those people healthy, they stood to make a profit. If they failed—and
patients needed hospitalization or expensive specialty care—
they stood to lose money.

These plans were touted as better in coordinating care for
low-income participants, but many states saw them simply as a
quick and easy way to control yearly costs.

The Medicaid managed-care experiment had mixed
results. Several of the for-profit companies that entered the field
found they could not make enough money in it and withdrew.
Interestingly, some public hospital systems created their own
managed Medicaid plans, again with mixed results depending
on the state's level of reimbursement in the first place. Atlanta's
Grady Memorial Hospital was one of them, although the plan
was abandoned after just a few years.

The Walmart Effect

Meanwhile, when reporters and health reform groups were able to get their hands on enrollment data coming for Medicaid and CHIP plans, they found that many kids covered by the taxpayer-subsidized plans were the children of low-wage earners working at large retailers, such as Walmart. Invariably, they worked for employers who relied on part-time workers and often offered health insurance only to managerial workers. (In thirteen states alone, Medicaid or a CHIP plan covered an estimated 55,000 Walmart employees or their children; more than 10,000 alone in Georgia's PeachCare for Kids program.)

The ensuing publicity prompted some of the large employers to start offering health coverage. The companies turned to the high-deductible, low-cost premium plans that were supposed to help with affordability for both the employer and the employee.

How well these incremental marketplace reform efforts worked is hard to measure. Individuals and families go in and out of insurance coverage, often within the same year, making the data from population surveys pretty spongy. Workers in new jobs sometimes have to wait three to six months before qualifying for coverage, taking a chance to live without it in the interim. Others, especially young, healthy adults, simply don't want to pay for it.

Going uninsured can be risky. A major accident, not covered by another form of insurance, or an unanticipated diagnosis of cancer, or even diabetes, could leave individuals and families thousands of dollars in debt, financially crippling them for years.

And, of course some adults—not an insignificant number by any means—couldn't get health insurance, even if they wanted it and were willing to pay for it. Because they had pre-existing medical conditions and were considered health risks, insurance companies estimated they would lose money on them, so they were denied coverage.

Still, this much we know:

During the debate over Hillarycare, an estimated 31 to 35 million Americans did not have insurance coverage, a number that represented approximately 14.8 percent of the country's population under sixty-five, the age of Medicare eligibility. By the time Barack Obama took office in early 2009, the percentage was 16.1.

The overall cost of care had not been contained, and the efforts at making insurance affordable had not moved the needle. Indeed, since the enactment of Medicare and Medicaid, more adult Americans than ever were living without health insurance, a number that was fast approaching fifty million people. Millions more held policies that forced them to pay thousands of dollars out of their own pockets before benefits would be paid. Others had cheap policies with poor benefits. Unpaid medical bills had become the leading cause of personal bankruptcy.

Support for a Comprehensive Plan Grows

Indeed, for the first time in polling history, a large majority (69 percent) of Americans surveyed by the Gallup organization said it was time for the federal government to guarantee coverage for all Americans. This set the stage for the presidential election of 2008 when health care once again became a major theme.

As discussed in the Introduction, the debate and passage of the Affordable Care Act in 2010, known and embraced by the new president as "Obamacare," was the most significant health care reform effort the nation has attempted in four decades.

The basics of the law most people know: Everyone is required to have insurance, or pay a fine. Depending on personal or family income, the federal government subsidizes the cost of premiums purchased on an insurance exchange run by the state, or by the federal government.

People who still cannot afford one of the plans may be eligible—depending on whether their state allows it—for Medicaid coverage, which was to be expanded up to a level of 138 percent of poverty (or $16,242 for an individual and $33,365 for a family of four under the 2015 poverty guidelines). Insurance companies can no longer screen out applicants with preexisting medical conditions for coverage under their plans. All plans available for purchase must contain a minimum benefit package that provides basic, preventive care services as well as covers the cost of hospitalization.

To hear the debate over the law then, and still today, you'd be forgiven for thinking that the federal government had assumed control of how medicine is practiced and paid for in the country. Yet the commercial insurance industry is still alive and well in the United States; physicians are busy teaming up to create new practice models; drug company profits remain high; and many American hospitals continue to expand and offer new services while others are merging with their one-time competitors. The private marketplace for health care is as robust as ever.

Still, despite news media and public-policy watchdogs declaring these repeated claims of a government takeover as "pants-on-fire" lies, the belief has taken hold in a sizable segment of the population. The mother of all ironies is that in more recent surveys—indeed, as Obamacare was being rolled out and more Americans were signing up for coverage—the majority opinion among the public (52 percent in a Gallup survey in late 2014) was that the federal government should not take on the responsibility of guaranteeing health coverage. The percentage of Americans who believed it was the federal government's role to do so had shrunk from 69 to 45 in the space of seven years.

The huge falloff in support of federal reform in late 2014 no doubt was related to the disastrous technical problems with the early rollout of the Obamacare insurance exchanges that year. It was also at this time when many Americans who already had private policies found out that those policies no longer met the minimum benefits standard, and they would have to find a new plan that did. This realization confirmed the worst fears of opponents of the law that the government was taking away their choice even though many would eventually sign up for more comprehensive coverage for close to the same costs.

The controversies sparked by the new law are also illustrative of how the country can't seem to settle on who is responsible for taking care of the poor. Moreover, a large segment of the Republican Party is simply opposed to any major role by the federal government in health care at all, even going so far as to suggest Medicare be privatized and Medicaid be abandoned in favor of direct grants to the states to create their own programs for the poor.

Ideological disagreements about the role of government in this country are not unusual; we've dealt with them in campaigns for years. But the logistics of health care reform, especially Obamacare, where states get to decide whether they wanted to create their own insurance exchanges and if they want to extend Medicaid coverage to more of the working poor, torqued the ideological division about health care more than ever.

Meanwhile, millions of Americans are left behind to fend for themselves in the costliest health care system on the planet. When they need help, they turn to public charity hospitals that must care for them.

As others have noted, Obamacare is not so much a national health reform policy as it is a tax and insurance regulation process for use by fifty different states to try to get more Americans covered by making insurance more affordable.

Not unexpectedly, after the first full year of the law in 2014, some states fared better than others. Those states that enacted their own health insurance exchanges and expanded Medicaid saw substantial reductions in the rate of uninsured. Kentucky, for instance, cut its rate of uninsured residents in half in the first year. Even states like Georgia, where political leaders publicly proclaimed they would act as obstructionists to the law, saw substantial reductions in the rate of uninsured thanks to the subsidies made available through the federal exchange.

NURSING HOMES AND THEIR CLOUT IN GEORGIA
Milking More Money from Washington

Late in 2014, Georgia ran into a problem with another financing scheme it used for Medicaid reimbursement. This time it was the mechanism the state used to get more federal money for nursing homes.

A few years earlier, the state had set up a bed tax for nursing homes similar to what it had done for hospitals. It was an accounting arrangement called "intergovernmental transfers" that allowed Georgia to draw down more federal matching funds for nursing homes to use. Only this scheme was set up for thirty-four nursing homes that were ostensibly owned by local government development authorities, even though they were managed by private firms or individuals.

By using intergovernmental transfers—supposedly taxes raised by the development authorities—these nursing homes could be paid at Medicare rates, much higher than the state would normally reimburse for services provided to Medicaid patients.

Around the country, the Centers for Medicare & Medicaid Services had been looking into the process to ensure that it was being carried out properly. And CMS cried foul when its investigation in Georgia showed that private owners, corporations, and a cash management group—not the government authorities—put up the state's share of the financing plan. Going back five years, federal taxpayers had sent Georgia nearly $200 million in overpayments to the state for these thirty-four nursing homes. Now the Feds wanted the money back.

Georgia officials disputed the federal investigation and refused to pay any of the money back. Refunding the money, the state said, "would result in unjust enrichment to the federal government," although it had been taxpayers in New Jersey, Utah, and virtually every other state who sent the money to Washington that Georgia had been improperly getting in the first place.

Despite the protestations, the state agreed to end the program in late 2014.

Nursing Homes and Hospitals

The 2015 Georgia general assembly refused to consider any measure that would have expanded Medicaid for the 500,000 to 600,000 Georgians who could be benefiting from it under the terms of the Affordable Care Act. Georgia's hospitals had been asking for the expansion for several years, pointing out that the federal government would cover 100 percent of the cost of expansion in 2014, 2015, and 2016. Rural hospitals, several of which were in danger of closing, could use the relief that covering more uninsured Georgians would provide them.

No deal, the state told the hospitals.

In contrast, the 2015 general assembly found a way to appropriate a $27 million rate increase for about forty nursing homes that they felt could use a little more, especially if most of the money came from Washington.

Lobbyists for the state's nursing home industry wanted the additional federal money so the new owners of these homes could make improvements to their facilities. State officials readily agreed.

There are about 290 nursing homes in Georgia compared to about 115 hospitals. Like public hospitals, they rely heavily on Medicaid to pay the bills for the elderly and disabled. Whenever it can, the state seems ready to help nursing homes out.

Why is this?

Local politics, mostly. Many of the state's independent nursing homes are owned by individuals in small towns and communities who know legislators firsthand, go to church with them, and break bread with them at civic group functions. Their social relationships are close and personal. Community hospitals, by contrast, are owned by government authorities or tied to regional health systems. Their administrators come and go.

It probably also helps that the state's nursing home owners always seem to be among the top leaders in campaign contributions to Georgia legislative candidates. Governor Nathan Deal's campaigns and political action committees backing his candidacy alone have received about $900,000 from nursing home interests. Former governors, Democrat and Republican, have felt the largesse of the industry over the years as well.

Hospitals, doctors, and health care groups are not shy about spreading their lobbying and campaign contributions around either. But there seems little question nursing homes get the better bang for what their bucks can buy in Georgia.

By the second quarter of 2015, the number of uninsured Americans had been reduced to about thirty-two million, down to the lowest level in fifteen years. Significantly, many of these newly insured were getting help from federal taxpayers who were subsidizing the new plans to make them affordable.

Yet in many states, especially in the South, millions of Americans had been excluded from this wave of health care reform. That's mostly the result of these states refusing to expand Medicaid eligibility, as envisioned under the law, but declared to be optional for the states by the Supreme Court decision of 2012.

These states purposely left behind about five million people, mostly adults working in low-wage jobs who can't afford private insurance even with a subsidy, but whose meager wages still make them ineligible for their state's Medicaid program. About half of these Americans live in three states—Texas, Florida, and Georgia—where Republican governors and legislators have steadfastly refused to consider expansion.

The refusal becomes all the more problematic for these states because of a provision of the 2010 law regarding the disproportionate share program that the federal government had been using to help hospitals that cared for large numbers of poor and uninsured patients. Under the ACA as approved by Congress, the disproportionate share program was supposed to end. The lawmakers reasoned that, with the new subsidized insurance exchanges and the expansion of Medicaid to the working poor, the need for the program would be diminished. But with the high court's decision that states could opt out of Medicaid expansion, all that changed.

Public hospitals like Grady as well as its counterparts in Florida, Texas, and other nonexpansion states—hospitals that serve a huge population of poor and uninsured—now faced a one-two punch to the gut. Not only would they not get Medicaid coverage for many of the poor they thought would be covered by the expansion, they risked losing the disproportionate share money to care for them. For Grady alone, the estimated loss was set at about $40 million per year, or about 5 percent of its operating budget.

Fortunately for them, the Obama administration and CMS (the Centers for Medicare & Medicaid Services) has adopted a go-slow attitude toward doing away with the disproportionate share funds. The threat of losing the money may have forced some Republican governors previously opposed to expansion to reconsider.

"Conscience" Gives Way to Ideology

Indeed, in 2013, Florida's Governor Rick Scott, a former executive and founder of a giant for-profit hospital corporation, got second thoughts about turning down billions of dollars in Medicaid expansion money offered through Obamacare. He could not "in good conscience deny the uninsured access to care," Scott said.

Like other Republican governors trying to find ways to get the federal funding, Scott had a plan. He proposed switching the state's Medicaid program over to management by private companies as a way toward ensuring fiscal discipline, while enrolling the estimated 900,000 Floridians who would have become eligible through expansion. The following year, the Florida state senate adopted a very similar plan in a 38-1 vote.

But Florida's Republican house leadership wasn't persuaded. They bottled the measure up in committee, and it got nowhere.

Scott's conscience about the uninsured hasn't seemed to bother him since his legislature rebuked him. More recently he has said he changed his mind again because the federal government can't be trusted to make good on its promise to pay most of the cost of Medicaid expansion.

In April of 2015, he said the state might sue the federal government if it doesn't agree to extend a $1 billion demonstration grant that helped hospitals and health clinics provide services to low-income people. Federal officials extended the money in 2014 for one more year when it appeared Florida was about to expand Medicaid. With the expansion, the demonstration grant would no longer be needed, the Feds said. Scott was furious. He called the federal response "coercion"—interestingly, the same word used by the US Supreme Court when it ruled mandatory Medicaid expansion unlawful.

This tug of war between Washington and state capitals is at the heart of how health care reform for poor people is managed in this country.

It is mostly a question of money. The goal is to get as much as possible from the Feds, while putting the bare minimum into such programs from the state treasury. It has been going on for years in the form of waivers and demonstration grants that states request—and often receive—from CMS for changes in how they run their Medicaid programs. Sometimes the waivers involve expansion of services; others may alter how the state raises its share of the cost of Medicaid services, or how the program is administered.

When Bill Clinton was governor of Arkansas, his administration got a waiver to expand Medicaid eligibility to cover pregnant uninsured women in the state. With the additional money, Arkansas made great progress in providing vital prenatal care to mothers who otherwise may not have been able to afford to get it. The expansion also helped improve the state's infant mortality rate. (Indeed, after Arkansas demonstrated success with the program, Medicaid adopted similar eligibility rules nationwide that states must follow.)

But more often, the interaction between the states and the federal government has less to do with expanding services for the poor than it does who pays for them. Many states have come to rely on special "uncompensated care" or "low-income pool" payment plans funded largely by the federal government to bolster their state Medicaid budgets.

The more recent debate in Florida is over a $1 billion low-income pool program that Scott demands the Feds continue to fund. Officials in Texas, Kansas, and Tennessee—all non-Medicaid-expansion states—are facing the potential loss of funding for similar programs that had originally been approved as temporary demonstration grants. California, Massachusetts, Arizona, Hawaii, and New Mexico have these programs in place too. But because they have expanded Medicaid, the impact on the state budget will not be nearly as substantial when the grants expire.

Another example in Georgia demonstrates well the politics of state spending for the poor. Opposition to the ACA is the bedrock position of the state's GOP leadership, so much so that they seem willing to surgically remove their noses to spite Obamacare's face.

Because of Georgia's consistently high poverty levels, federal taxpayers have always provided about two-thirds of the cost of Medicaid in the state. The rest is the responsibility of Georgia's taxpayers and the people they elect to statewide office. Yet in recent decades, going back to Democratic Party rule, before Republicans gained control in 2002, Georgia's general assembly has not kept pace in appropriating the amount of state money needed to provide care for the hundreds of thousands of residents covered by the program.

In an attempt to minimize its own costs, Georgia did what other states have traditionally done—shortchanged hospitals and doctors who provide services for patients covered by Medicaid by paying them much less than what they would get for patients covered by private insurance or Medicare. For years, doctors and hospitals decried the low payments (and slow payments) they got from the state, but the process was entirely legal under Medicaid financing.

That's because the federal government determines how much providers are paid only for Medicare services. For Medicaid, that determination is made by the individual states.

(This, despite the fact that most of the money going into state Medicaid programs is coming from the US Treasury.)

Still, stingy reimbursement for Medicaid didn't always work, and the cost of Medicaid to Georgia's annual budgets continued to climb inexorably.

This led to bitter complaints from state leaders that Medicaid was crowding out what they believe is more worthy state spending on budget necessities such as transportation, education, prisons, and economic development. Even during the relatively healthy economic years of 2002 to 2007, the state clamped down on Medicaid spending, saying providers needed to understand the need for austerity in the budget process.

By 2010, the year Congress was debating and approving Obamacare, it was obvious to Georgia's political leadership that lowballing Medicaid reimbursements would not be enough. So the general assembly enacted a first-of-its-kind "bed tax" on the state's hospitals to raise additional revenue for Medicaid.

Like other financing schemes they created, the state promised hospitals that the additional money would be used to draw down more federal dollars into the state Medicaid program—roughly $2 for every $1 the state put up. The additional money could in turn be sent back to most of them in the form of higher payments under the disproportionate share program. (Georgia is one of those states where most of its hospitals are deemed to be above average when it comes to providing charity care.)

To get the state out of its self-created financial hole, hospitals put a little money in—1.45 percent of their net patient revenue—but most of them would get more back than what they actually contributed. (Largely unspoken during the debate was that the hospitals could simply shift the cost of the bed tax to patients with insurance, which meant that the state's insured residents were effectively subsidizing the scheme.)

To soften the impact, state leaders estimated the tax would only be necessary for a few years, just to get the state program back on track. And it would likely mean no further reductions in reimbursement levels.

But three years later, as the economic recession continued to take its toll, Georgia was still in financial trouble. The US Supreme Court ruled the year before that states had the option to reject expansion under Obamacare, and there was no talk at all about opening up eligibility in Georgia. Georgia wanted to limit state spending on the existing Medicaid program, which still faced a $700 million shortfall in caring for the now 1.7 million residents who depended on it.

Georgia's hospitals were given a choice in 2013: renew the tax or face a new 20 percent reduction in the payments they would get for taking care of Medicaid patients—a rate that already was less than the actual cost of those services. The hospitals agreed.

The renewed tax did not erase the state's Medicaid deficit. It helped, but it still came up several hundred million dollars short. State legislators left their session in 2013 exhausted by the debate over Medicaid. The idea of expanding Medicaid as envisioned by the ACA had never even surfaced.

A Question of Priorities

What makes this anecdote doubly ironic is that the following year there finally was a debate in the Georgia general assembly about Medicaid expansion. Having settled the bed tax issue the year before, health care advocates believed Georgia might finally consider expansion in 2014.

Governor Nathan Deal, an outspoken Republican critic of Obamacare, was up for reelection. Some thought he would perhaps be more open to expansion once he cleared his party's primary where he was facing extreme right-wing opposition that condemned any talk of it. Plus, in the November election, Deal would face a young state senator, Jason Carter—the grandson of former President Jimmy Carter—who would almost certainly move to expand Medicaid if he won.

Around the country, several other Republican governors were seeing the wisdom of getting 100 percent federal funding for expanding the program to individuals making up to 138 percent of the poverty line. (The ACA promised complete federal funding for the first three years and no less than 90 percent funding in subsequent years.)

Economic impact analysis in these states, as well as in Georgia, showed that the cost of expansion was more than eclipsed by shoring up the bottom lines of hospitals as well as saving thousands of health care industry jobs. Moreover, it would provide a significant boost to the state's small rural hospitals, about a dozen of which were in danger of closing because they could not sustain additional losses in uncompensated care. This is why many predicted Deal might change his mind after reelection in 2014 and find a way to expand Medicaid in 2015.

They couldn't have been more wrong.

Instead, what the Georgia general assembly did was pass a law in 2014 that took that decision out of the governor's hands. The new law, signed by Deal, declared that only the general assembly could expand Medicaid eligibility, an action that in most states can be taken by the executive branch.

If Deal had any inkling of expansion after reelection—he easily defeated Carter, who decided not to make Medicaid expansion a major campaign theme—it evaporated with the general assembly's action. Instead, he declared Medicaid too costly for the state and criticized it as ineffective. His evidence for that was that most Georgia doctors refused to take Medicaid patients. He failed to mention that the state had been shortchanging them in reimbursements for years.

Besides, he said, a new Congress and a new president may repeal the ACA after the 2016 elections and give the states what they really need: block grant funding to design their own health care programs for the poor. (He said the same thing prior to the 2012 election, and again in 2014.) For Deal, this next-election-could-change-everything-theme has become a boilerplate response to inquiries about Medicaid expansion.

Interestingly, about 100,000 additional Georgians enrolled in Medicaid anyway in 2014 under the existing eligibility standards—adults in Georgia must earn less than 34 percent of the poverty level to be eligible for coverage. The federal government will continue to pay about 65 percent of the cost of their care, which means Georgia budget makers will have to find a way to pay the state's portion for the coverage of these new additions to the Medicaid rolls.

It is unlikely that the state's political leadership will enact any kind of tax increase—even on cigarettes, liquor, or other easier targets—to pay for these additional enrollees. Nor, if there is a Democrat in the White House, will they be able to continue to create financing schemes like the bed tax ploy. Once again, they may have to turn to shortchanging hospitals for their care of Medicaid patients. All this could happen as the federal officials shut off funding, as planned, for the disproportionate share program—the financial lifeblood for rural and urban public hospitals in nonexpansion states.

Had Medicaid been expanded in the state the way Obamacare was envisioned, an additional 500,000 to 600,000 Georgians could have been enrolled, with the federal government paying for 100 percent of their coverage. By refusing to expand Medicaid, Georgia was leaving about $9 million a day on the table, unclaimed for use by the neediest people in the state and the hospitals that treat them.

Why So Many Are Left Behind

Diving this deep into this one state's decision-making about Medicaid is illustrative, not just as a political narrative about how warped the Obamacare fight has become, but because it speaks to priorities.

When pressed to go beyond his boilerplate responses about Medicaid, Georgia's governor and his aides will say that the program is "simply unaffordable" and, if the federal government ever reneged on its portion of financing, would be a catastrophe for the state. Yet Georgia has a $21 billion annual budget. Medicaid expansion would cost state taxpayers an estimated $200 to $400 million yearly, a significant amount, to be certain, but not an unaffordable one.

Nor do there seem to be similar concerns about federal untrustworthiness to finance other long-standing state and federally financed programs such as transportation, education, and economic development. The state has never considered turning down federal money in those areas.

What sets Medicaid apart from these other important programs is clear: Medicaid is designed to assist the poor. In Georgia, and unfortunately in too many other states, history shows that assisting the poor is simply not a priority.

Wayne Flynt, professor emeritus at Auburn University and a respected historian, has made a career writing about Southern states and their shortsightedness in addressing poverty, especially the connection between health and school performance.

"They are clearly related," Flynt said. "Children who suffer from chronic health problems have more trouble in school." They often grow up to be "unhealthy employees who reduce productivity and raise insurance rates" for the businesses that hire them, which in turn suppresses economic opportunity in the state.

While researching a book recently, Flynt said, he found Alabama ranked forty-ninth in obesity, diabetes, high blood pressure, and child poverty; forty-eighth in infant mortality; forty-sixth in heart disease; forty-third in strokes; and forty-second in smoking and cancer.

Statistics like these reflect "a stunning lack of vision, leadership and courage among [Alabama's] elites," he wrote in an opinion piece in 2014.

This reliance on the states to implement and help pay for programs aimed at assisting the poor is the primary reason why so many Americans are left behind in our health care system. It also is why the nation's public hospitals that care for them fail to thrive.

THE AMERICAN INSURANCE CHECKERBOARD

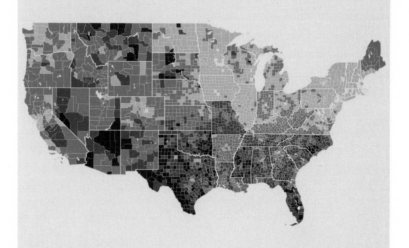

2015 Uninsured Rates

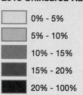

	0% - 5%
	5% - 10%
	10% - 15%
	15% - 20%
	20% - 100%

2015 Uninsured Estimates: This interactive map shows the 2015 uninsured rates by county across the United States. *[Enroll America map used with permission. To look closer at the changes at the state and county level between 2013 and 2015 Enroll America's interactive map can be accessed at https://www.enrollamerica.org/research-maps/maps/changes-in-uninsured-rates-by-county/#]*

If you are poor or not covered on the job, where you live in America has a lot to do with whether you have access to health insurance to cover you when you get sick.

Over the last several years, Enroll America has created a series of maps showing the projected percentage of uninsured residents of every county in the U.S. The health advocacy group uses Census surveys and other data points to keep track of the states and counties where lack of access to insurance is most critical.

When the group issued its 2015 map and compared it to 2013, prior to the full implementation of the Patient Protection and Accountable Care Act, the results were stunning.

In 2013, many counties in the U.S. had uninsurance rates above 15 percent. In some parts of the South, one in four adult residents did not have insurance coverage.

By 2015, after nearly two full years of the new law, the percentage of uninsured had dropped precipitously around the country. Among Northeastern and Midwestern states, the rates in some counties dipped below five percent. Most were well below ten percent.

But in the South and a handful of other states outside the region, the picture was much different. Even in these states the rates were in decline, but not nearly as fast as elsewhere in the country.

The reason: Most of the states in the South have refused to expand Medicaid coverage to low-income adults who would have been covered under the law had the U.S. Supreme Court not ruled in 2012 that Medicaid expansion was optional. The 2015 Enroll America map, reproduced here, shows the results of that refusal. Arkansas stands out among the Southern states because it expanded Medicaid access. Many counties in

Arkansas had their rates cut in half thanks to the new law. Otherwise, the rural South is still awash with people who don't have health insurance. Most rural southern counties have rates well above ten percent, many still above fifteen percent.

The three most populous states in the South, Texas, Florida and Georgia, now have the highest number, and the highest rate of uninsured residents in the U.S.

Without Medicaid expansion, public hospitals in these and other states will have to continue to provide care to poor and low-income adults on a charity basis whereas their counterparts in expansion states are now being paid for their services.

(NOTE: Louisiana's new governor has said he will implement Medicaid expansion later in 2016. Alabama's governor is said to favor expansion as well.)

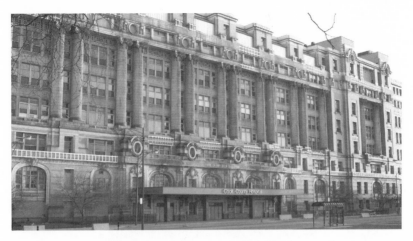

The old Cook County Hospital in Chicago was the backdrop for several motion pictures and television series, including The Fugitive and E.R. But its history can be traced back to 1832 when the state of Illinois assigned the care of "pauper patients" to county governments. The beaux-arts structure on Harrison Drive was built in 1916 and became the site of the nation's first blood bank and numerous other medical innovations. Through most of its years, County became the subject of investigations into public corruption and patronage, but it also developed a reputation as a great teaching hospital that was committed to serving the poor. In 2002 it shut its doors when the new John H. Stroger Jr. Hospital of Cook County opened just down the street. Like Charity in New Orleans, old County hospital in Chicago remains vacant. *(Photo credit: Jeff Dahl, 2008, Cook County Hospital, Wikimedia Commons, CC-SA)*

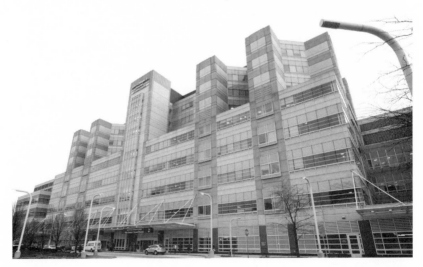

The John H. Stroger Jr. Hospital is part of a massive Cook County health and hospital system that no longer has to bear all the burden of indigent care by itself. In recent years, County has embarked on a program called CountyCare, which functions as an HMO-style insurance plan for county residents on Medicaid. The new program is credited for greatly enhancing County's financial performance and is being touted as a model for other urban systems around the country. *(Photo courtesy of Cook County Health & Hospitals System)*

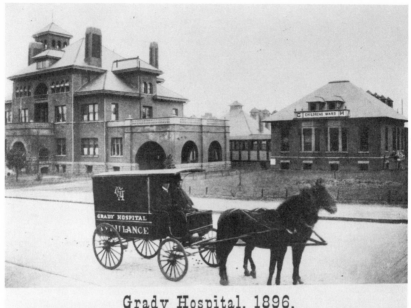

Grady Hospital, 1896.

Grady Memorial Hospital in Atlanta opened in 1892 with about half of its cost paid for by the city and the rest donated by local individuals and charities. By 1896 the hospital had a separate children's ward and its own horse-drawn ambulance. *(Photo courtesy of Special Collections and Archives, Georgia State University Library)*

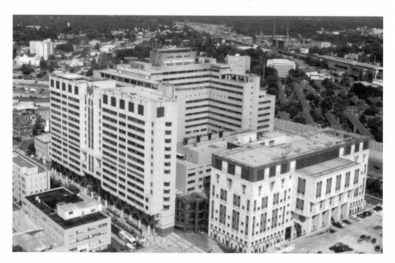

The modern Grady Hospital opened its doors in 1958 and still maintained racially separate wings – one on each side of the oldest part of the building in the center of this photo. Around the time Medicare was enacted in 1965 the hospital was forced to desegregate. In the 1990s the hospital was renovated and expanded to include outpatient clinics and new specialized treatment centers. But the renovation project went over budget, leaving two floors on one wing of the hospital unfinished. (They have since been built out with the help of private foundation money.) *(Photo © Grady Health System)*

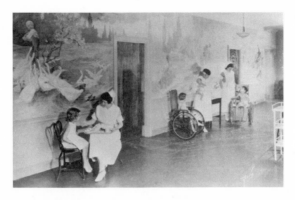

During the Great Depression artists working through New Deal agencies were dispatched to public buildings, including hospitals, to create murals, sculptures, and other public works. One such mural was on the wall of the children's ward of the old Grady Hospital in Atlanta. *(Photo © Atlanta History Center)*

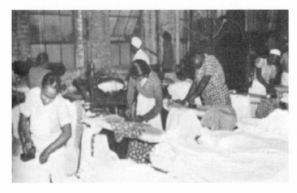

In 1940, the hospital's main laundry room was staffed almost exclusively by black women. *(Photo © Grady Health System)*

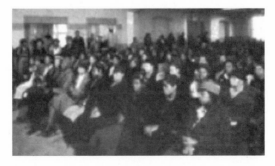

Almost from its opening in 1892, Grady Memorial Hospital had racially segregated facilities, including separate waiting rooms. This is the waiting from for black patients in 1936. The segregation led many people in the city to refer to the hospital as "the Gradys." *(Photo © Grady Health System)*

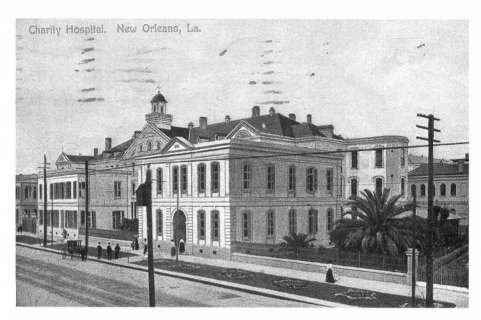

The original Charity Hospital in New Orleans opened in 1736, a gift of French seaman and boat builder Jean Louis and staffed by the Sisters of Charity. Through storms and deadly outbreaks of yellow fever, Charity stood as a New Orleans institution and landmark. This 1909 postcard depicts the Charity Hospital that was built in 1832 and served the city for more than 100 years. *(Photo credit: Wikimedia Creative Commons, postcard dated 12 November, 1909)*

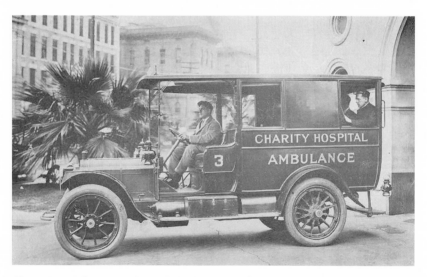

Charity Hospital in New Orleans also had its own ambulance service as shown in this photo from a 1912 annual report. *(Photo credit: Internet Archive Book Images, Ambulance, Charity Hospital, New Orleans, Louisiana (1912), Wikimedia CC-SA)*

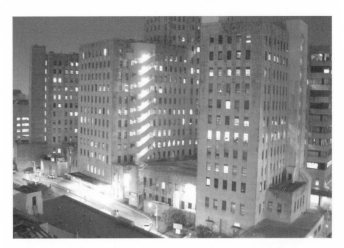

The art deco fortress that most of us came to know as Charity Hospital was built in 1939 and was one of the nation's largest Public Works Administration projects. This night photo of the bustling facility was taken less than two weeks before Hurricane Katrina hit New Orleans in 2005, flooding the basement and emergency room. Despite the damage caused by the breach of the city's levee system, Charity could have been up and running again in a matter of weeks, according to disaster assistance officials. But the state of Louisiana, which owned the hospital, decided to padlock the gates, closing the book on perhaps the most iconic public hospital in the country. It remains vacant. *(Photo credit: Niels Olson [CC BY-SA 2.0 via Wikimedia Commons])*

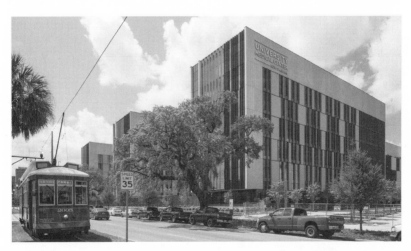

With a large dose of federal disaster assistance money, the new University Medical Center of New Orleans opened in 2015 around the 10th anniversary of Hurricane Katrina. Much smaller than Charity, the UMC is the city's acute care facility for indigent patients. The new hospital is part of the LSU health system, which has strong ties to other hospitals in the city and a network of primary care clinics that Charity lacked. Public health advocates in the city and state are watching closely to see whether UMC has the same level of dedication to charity care as the hospital it replaced. *(Photo credit: NBBJ/Sean Airhart, courtesy University Medical Center of New Orleans)*

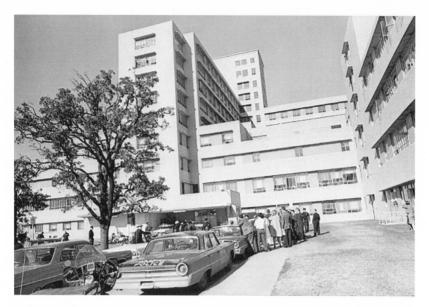

Perhaps best known as the hospital where President John F. Kennedy, Jr. was pronounced dead after his assassination (see above), Parkland Memorial Hospital in Dallas is also one of the largest public hospitals in Texas. In 2015, Parkland opened a state-of-the-art, $1.3 billion facility with the help of a major bond issue approved by local voters (see below). But because the state of Texas has refused to expand Medicaid to more of the working poor, Parkland will need to rely on local taxpayer support to offset the cost of care to uninsured patients. *(Photo © Getty Images. Mourning at Parkland, by Art Rickerby)*

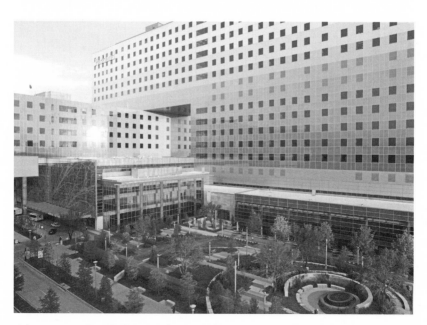

(Photo courtesy of Parkland Health & Hospital System)

PART II
ESSENTIAL PLACES

Tracie Steadman knew almost instantly that the procedure was a success.

Hours earlier she had suffered a stroke at her home outside of Atlanta. While she remained conscious, she couldn't move her right arm and had no feeling on the right side of her body. Thankfully, her husband knew the warning signs and called 911.

After an evaluation in the ER, she was rushed to one of the neuroscience procedure rooms at Grady Memorial Hospital, where Dr. Raul Nogueira snaked a tiny catheter deep into the arteries of her brain.

Nogueira, a world-class interventional neurologist from Brazil recruited to practice at Grady by the Emory University School of Medicine, asked Tracie, who was awake and on the table, how she was doing.

"I could move my arm and hand and wave at him," she said. "I knew as soon as he got it."

Nogueira had used what was just a few years earlier an investigational device, but now is the gold standard of care, to find and remove a stubborn blot clot in the brain that didn't respond to conventional blood thinners and other stroke therapies.

Guided by live-action, detailed images of his patient's arteries displayed on a monitor in front of him, Nogueira pushed the device to the site of the obstruction and literally snatched the clot away, opening blood flow once again to the region of the brain that controls movement and other vital body functions.

Not that long ago, a clot that couldn't be dissolved with targeted blood thinners would have rendered Tracie at least partially paralyzed and in need of long-term physical rehabilitation, if she was lucky enough to survive. Instead, three days after being admitted to Grady's ER, she was out of the hospital, physically fine and unencumbered in any significant way by the stroke she had just endured.

Like many other patients at the hospital, Tracie had no insurance to cover her care at Grady. She had been laid off about 18 months earlier from a human services job with the local YMCA—a good job that had provided full coverage for the ten years she worked there. It was the longest she had ever been without a job or insurance, and the pressure she was experiencing around the same time—losing her house, declaring bankruptcy, separating from her husband, and dealing with a son who was diagnosed with schizophrenia—clearly had taken a toll.

She was feeling stressed, but thought she could handle it. Besides, she said, without insurance she couldn't really afford to go to a doctor.

Tracie credits Grady's neuroscience center for not just saving her life, but getting her recentered on things that really matter, such as reconciling with her husband, helping her son, writing poetry, and sharing it with others.

She works at the hospital's stroke center now. Most days you can find her behind a small desk in the waiting room, making sure families understand what is happening to their loved ones and getting their questions answered. She educates people about the risks and warning signs of stroke, and she is vigilant about keeping track of her blood pressure, cholesterol, and blood sugar levels and other known contributors to the condition.

"I feel like I can give them something to help them through this. It is so scary at times," she said. "Anything that makes them smile. I can give them a hug, recite some poetry for them, bring them some lunch from the cafeteria—anything to give something back for the gift I was given by the people who took such great care of me."

Cardiovascular disease—and stroke in particular—is a chronic medical problem for African-Americans and other minorities in the United States. The fact that African-Americans die from stroke at overall rates significantly higher than whites has been well established for decades.

But what is less well known is the staggering toll stroke takes among African-Americans in their forties and fifties, like Tracie Steadman. Blacks between the ages of forty-five and sixty-four have a mortality rate from stoke that is three times what it is for whites. Moreover, many of those who survive are so disabled that they cannot work or require long-term care.

Most poor or uninsured African-American stroke victims don't have access to the gold standard of care that Tracie Steadman found at Grady. And, even more problematic, the racial disparity of access and treatment for almost all other chronic, debilitating conditions that afflict poor and minority Americans is not just limited to stroke.

Indeed, the most damning indictment of America's $3 trillion health care system is that the marvelous strides it has made toward diagnosing and treating chronic diseases are not equally shared among its people.

The United States as an Outlier

What makes physicians, public health experts, and even ordinary citizens in other countries when they hear about it shake their heads in disbelief is how the US system that spends so much on health care can fare so poorly when measuring disease, disability, and death "outcomes" in comparison to the rest of the world.

Why is it that life expectancy among Americans remains below eighty years and lags badly behind Japan, Italy, France,

Canada, the United Kingdom, and forty-three other nations? Why, as well, do we spend on average nearly $8,000 per year per person on health care while France spends, on average, half of that?

Life expectancy by race within our own country raises even more troubling questions. Consider that there is an astounding twenty-five-year difference between the life expectancy of Asian-American women and African-American men living in the United States. The former can expect to live, on average, 86.7 years, while the latter live just 61.7. What accounts for that?

The generally accepted answer to this has always been that the gap between rich and poor in our country—a gap that is much broader and more enduring than other wealthy countries—explains much of the disparity. And because there is a higher prevalence of poverty among African-Americans and Latinos, for instance, that could explain why, as a group, they don't live as long as whites or Asians.

Often unspoken in this discussion, but still a common stereotype, is that the poor simply don't take care of themselves; they eat nonnutritious meals and don't get enough exercise. They drink too much alcohol. The women don't get enough exercise and become obese. The men engage in risky, violent behavior.

There's nothing wrong with our system that better patients won't cure. In other words: it's not the system, it's them.

This same explanation has even been employed to explain why babies die in their first year of life in the United States at rates much higher than the rates in Great Britain, France, and Japan.

Even though the US mortality rate has improved in recent years, it remains embarrassingly much higher for minority babies than it is for whites. The national rate would fall in line with other countries if low-income and poor women would take care of themselves during pregnancy, or so the claim is often heard.

Often left out of these explanations is that it might be the income gap itself—the difference between having enough money to purchase insurance and health care and being so poor you can purchase neither—that accounts for most of the difference. In virtually all other countries that we should compare ourselves against, there is universal access to health insurance and health care as an entitlement of citizenship.

The simple fact is that our country has yet to fully embrace that notion, except for the elderly, who are entitled to Medicare when they reach the age of sixty-five. We've carved out some exceptions along the way, creating, for instance, coverage for kidney failure in the Medicare program, regardless of age or income levels. And poor women who wouldn't otherwise qualify for Medicaid can get care if they get pregnant, as can their babies. But these are exceptions to the general rule that able-bodied, nonelderly Americans are on their own when it comes to health care.

There have been some unintended marketplace consequences from even these limited efforts to expand coverage—consequences that have made running America's large public hospitals more difficult and increased the burdens placed upon them.

We have no comprehensive plan for covering the chronic health problems that beset Americans without insurance. We force our uninsured, low-income citizens to ration spending on medical care against all their other necessities.

And our health care outcomes show it.

Many Americans still steadfastly believe that poor people can get free care when they need it by simply going to an emergency room. Even President George W. Bush, as late as 2007, declared that Americans need not worry about their fellow citizens not having health insurance because hospital ERs will take them in when they need help.

Not so much.

Hospital ERs are required to take in a patient whose condition is so unstable as to be immediately life threatening, which is why everyone is supposed to get a cursory screening when they come through the door. Many American hospitals will provide a responsible level of free care for those who show up sick and in need of help, even those without insurance.

But it is a widely accepted practice, and entirely legal, for nonprofit and private hospitals to send patients without life-threatening conditions who come to their ERs to a public hospital for what they deem to be nonemergency care.

You need only walk into an emergency room of any large public hospital in the United States to confirm this. There you will find people in need of basic medical care for dozens of chronic conditions such as hypertension, diabetes, cancer, chest pain from heart disease, and depression and for whom the public hospital is their only source of health care.

Public Hospitals and the American Safety Net

This one defining characteristic of American medicine—that we don't share our medical wealth equally—is why public hospitals exist and why they matter. Amazingly, most of them do quite well in taking care of the immediate needs of their patients by turning them over to experts in specialty fields backed up by fellows in training as well as by resident physicians rotating through the hospital.

The quality of care in some large public hospitals, especially those with a teaching component in specialty fields, can be second to none in a community.

Grady, for instance, can boast the best stroke care in Atlanta. Tracie Steadman is alive and well thanks to it. In fact, since the Joint Commission, a voluntary group that accredits hospitals in the United States started pushing for higher standards of stroke care a decade ago, public hospitals have led the way toward receiving advanced certification in stroke treatment. Yet, most privately insured patients wouldn't go near a charity hospital like Grady for stroke care.

Disparities aside, what happens when poor patients are discharged is as important as the care they get inside the hospital. And here is where the income and insurance gap can create havoc. Who pays for the prescription drugs that the uninsured need to stay well? Where will they go for follow-up care? How will they get to that free clinic halfway across town?

Failure to coordinate follow-up care often triggers a vortex of patient decline, a return trip to the emergency room, and readmission—the so-called frequent-flyer syndrome endemic among the poor at public hospitals around the country.

In the worst-case scenarios, it can lead to premature death. At least five African-American women a day die from breast cancer due to the disparities in how they are diagnosed and treated compared to white women, according to a 2014 Avon Foundation study of breast cancer treatment in large American cities.

As they have been forced to do since they were created, public hospitals are working on ways to deal with these disparities, even if they face uncertain funding from government sources for their efforts.

It's also worth noting that the problems outlined here are most acutely felt in the South, where the poverty rate is significantly higher than other regions of the country and where state Medicaid programs have been unusually restrictive when it comes to enrollment and how much they pay doctors and hospitals to provide care for those lucky enough to be enrolled.

Medicaid in the South

One compelling statistic among Southern states stands out.

In 2014, 61 percent of those enrolled in Southern state Medicaid programs were children; 49 percent were adults. For the rest of the country, Medicaid enrollment is almost a reverse image—on average about 70 percent of those covered by Medicaid in the Northeast, Midwest, and West are adults, and 30 percent are children. In the South, if you are an able-bodied adult with no children—even if you don't have a job or any source of income—you are probably not eligible for Medicaid.

The Affordable Care Act of 2010 was supposed to deal with this by expanding Medicaid to millions of Americans who made too much money to qualify for it in the past, but not enough to afford private insurance. But most Southern states have refused to go along with the expansion.

Moreover, the ACA specifically excludes noncitizens from its benefits, which means that immigrants in the country illegally, and their children who were born elsewhere, but who can legally attend school here, cannot get insurance coverage through either Medicaid or the subsidized government exchanges. That fact alone leaves an estimated seven to nine million people living and often working in this country on their own, without health care coverage.

Hospitals like Grady in Atlanta, Jackson Memorial in Miami, Parkland in Dallas, and others must tackle these challenges. They do not get much help from their state "partners" in the jointly funded federal and state Medicaid programs; nor does there seem to be a lot of willingness by their nonprofit and private community competitors to take on more of the burden. That's understandable, given all the other changes that ACA has generated in the marketplace to make hospitals more efficient and to hold down costs.

America's large public hospitals do not have that option. They must respond to the patients who show up, regardless of ability to pay. But they also must adapt to changes in health policy, many of which, like the ACA, have fallen significantly short in dealing with the problem.

Many of them nevertheless excel at the challenge. The technology, expertise, and follow-up care given to Tracie Steadman at Grady is the best in Atlanta. Tracie believes Grady saved her life and provided her a second chance to accomplish the goals she had before her stroke.

But it should be noted, as well, that the quality of Tracie's care might not have been available if Grady had relied on state or local tax dollars to improve its neuroscience facilities. It took a private foundation to do that.

7

BRIDGING THE GAP BETWEEN THE RACES

The neonatal intensive care unit on the fifth floor of Grady Memorial Hospital can seem deceptively small. It spans the length of a football field, but none of the thirty to forty babies being cared for there on any given day are more than a few steps away from the nurses and specialist physicians who staff it around the clock.

It's a busy place. Nurses shuttle along the open corridors pushing laptop computers affixed to tables that can be raised or lowered as needed. Everything about the baby's condition— vital signs like heart rate, respiration, and temperature—is displayed at the bedside and can be transmitted via computer to the nurses. Equipment sounds are kept to a minimum, but there are still frequent bleeps from monitors and air pulses from ventilators heard around the room.

The babies stay in what used to be called incubators— clear plastic-walled isolation chambers where the inside temperature, oxygen levels, and light can be controlled. Nurses and parents alike can slide their hands and arms into gloves sewn into the sides so they can touch the infants without contaminating the isolette.

Most of the babies in the Grady NICU go there because they are extremely premature at birth, many weighing less than 1,500 grams, or 3.3 pounds.

Grady's NICU is reflective of the hospital's patient demographic mix. The vast majority of the babies are African-American. But unlike adult patients in the rest of the hospital, Medicaid usually covers the NICU babies. There are some privately insured babies there too—often born elsewhere and brought by special air and ground ambulances to Grady, which for many years in the 1970s and 1980s had the only fully equipped neonatal ICU in the northern half of Georgia.

The goal, said Dr. Bill Sexson, an Emory neonatologist who has run the unit for years, is to provide a mechanical atmosphere for the baby that closely resembles what he or she would have—should have—received in their mother's womb. The emphasis is on nutrition and respiration, providing food and oxygen for growth and organ development, especially for the baby's brain.

Between thirty-five to thirty-eight weeks of gestation, a baby's brain goes through a remarkable growth spurt—almost three milligrams a minute, but only if it is getting the oxygen it needs, Dr. Sexson said. That means the baby's lungs must be working properly, or supported carefully by mechanical means. If the baby is unable to eat, nutrition is supplied by special IV fluids that contain protein, fats, carbohydrates and minerals.

Medicine has made tremendous strides in recent decades in mechanical support of low-birth-weight infants cared for in the nation's NICUs. After years of dismal statistics, the nation's infant mortality rate, which is measured as the rate of 1,000 babies born alive who die in the first year of life, improved significantly between 1975 and 2000, reached a plateau for a few years, and eventually declined to 5.96 in 2013.

The mortality rate among black babies also improved significantly during this period, but it remains high—twice the rate compared to whites. Year to year those numbers fluctuate somewhat, but the disparity between black and white infant mortality remains one of the nation's most acute public health issues.

By some measures, the success the United States has achieved at reducing its infant mortality rate is as much the result of "saving" tiny babies in the NICU as it is in providing prenatal care and education of young mothers so they won't deliver prematurely in the first place.

We know this because the rate of low-birth-weight babies

in this country—those born weighing less than 2,500 grams (about 5.5 pounds), as well as those even smaller (1,500 grams or 3.3 pounds)—has not diminished significantly when compared to the overall improvement in infant mortality. Too many babies are still being born too soon and too small, but we have gotten highly skilled at getting many of them through their first year of life.

That was at least partially the goal of public-policy changes in the 1980s and 1990s that recognized poor pregnant women and their babies should have more accessible care than they had been getting up until that time and especially those who had the least: black women.

New eligibility rules allowed for easier enrollment in Medicaid for low-income pregnant women who prior to that would have fallen above income limits. Under these new directives, poor, pregnant women showing up at American hospitals ready to deliver could be covered under "presumptive" eligibility for Medicaid, even if the hospitals didn't get paid for taking care of them for months after having their babies.

More than just a sense of nobility informed these policy changes. If poor women could get coordinated care from the start of their pregnancies, they were less likely to deliver too early, and their babies would not need the expensive services of a NICU.

But, from a policy perspective, expanding Medicaid eligibility to pregnant women turned out to have some unintended consequences.

One of these was cost.

Caring for a baby born weighing 1,000 grams (about 2.2 pounds) or less in a NICU can run over $250,000. And with advances in neonatal technology, about 95 percent of these tiny babies now survive to their first birthday. (One hundred years ago, the mortality rate for babies that small was 95 percent—the reverse of what it is now.)

Unfortunately, very-low-birth-weight babies are also at much higher risk for cerebral palsy, seizure disorders, blindness, deafness, and learning disorders. This means they may need medical care for chronic conditions the rest of their lives.

By contrast, the best way to prevent early births is with consistent prenatal care for the mother. Inexpensive blood tests and screenings at the first prenatal visit can predict gestational diabetes, hypertension, and other maternal disorders that can be treated to reduce the risk that the baby will be delivered early. Spending $400 to $500 for taxpayer-financed prenatal care over nine months beats $4,000 to $5,000 a day for charges incurred in the NICU, followed by a lifetime of debilitation.

This is precisely why health advocates and public officials in states with high infant mortality rates pushed to expand Medicaid in the first place in order to get more low-income women into prenatal care through the program.

But, as a practical matter, something else happened.

Hospitals stood to recoup some of their indigent care costs by making sure pregnant women showing up in the ER when they were ready to deliver got enrolled in Medicaid. They moved aggressively to participate in the expansion and created social work teams to help the new mothers get all their paperwork for eligibility forms ready to go to the state before they were discharged. But most of these hospitals didn't provide prenatal care.

Unfortunately, many private-practice obstetricians, who would have provided the most cost-effective prenatal care for the same group of women, didn't get with the program. Many continued to deny care to low-income women, thinking that trying to get adequate reimbursement from state Medicaid programs for the prenatal care they provided was not worth the effort. Instead, they directed them to public hospitals and public health clinics, where they were unlikely to see the same health professional twice during their prenatal visits.

(To be fair, there are some excellent public health programs around the country for prenatal care, and they are often staffed by certified nurse practitioners and other highly qualified medical professionals. Some of them have visiting nurses who go to see pregnant women in their homes. These demonstration programs showed the effectiveness of consistent prenatal care in preventing low-birth-weight deliveries and complications during pregnancy. But, probably because of up-front costs, they were not widely adopted.)

Still, with this new payment source, hospitals in the 1980s and 1990s began to expand their nurseries, and more of them opened NICUs to accommodate a whole new group of patients. While Medicaid rates for labor and delivery for these newly eligible mothers fell short of what they got for patients with private insurance, it was better than nothing, which was what they were getting before. And it greatly expanded the options for low-income and uninsured women who no longer had to go to public hospitals to have their babies.

Moreover, even if their babies were somewhat premature, the NICUs in these hospitals could usually provide adequate care. If there was a more significant problem, the baby could be transferred to a higher-level NICU, usually one at a public hospital nearby.

Once again, it's easy to see how a major health care policy change aimed at the poor, while well intentioned, can sometimes backfire on the very institutions chartered to care for the poor in the first place.

Without an emphasis on getting low-income women adequate access to prenatal care and not just enrolling them in Medicaid and presuming they will find a doctor or clinic to provide it, a substantial portion of them will go without it and run the risk of delivering babies that are born too soon and need the costly services of a high-level NICU.

In a 2013 report on health disparities and inequality, the CDC concluded that preventing premature birth is the most important step the country could take to reduce the infant mortality gap among whites, blacks, and other racial and ethnic minorities.

Until then, neonatal units like the one at Grady will continue to be pressed into service caring for very-low-birth-weight babies whose mothers received inadequate or no prenatal care.

The hospital's outpatient clinics also routinely provide prenatal care and well-baby care for women on Medicaid and their children, but Grady remains the go-to hospital for too many poor Atlanta women who are pregnant and about to deliver. Other hospitals have picked up some of Grady's premature-baby patient load, but the tiniest babies and the ones with the most complications still end up there.

Kidney Disease: An All-American Story

Eduardo Agatone and his adult daughter, Christina, walked along Decatur Street in downtown Atlanta searching for a place for him to get kidney dialysis. It had been nearly a week since his last treatment, and his daughter knew waiting much longer would jeopardize his health.

Recent settlers in the Atlanta area, they had entered the country illegally through Texas and moved in with his brother in the suburb of Tucker. (Eduardo's last name was changed for this story.) His family told him that Grady Hospital would provide the service for free for anyone who needs it.

But they were misinformed. Grady stopped providing outpatient dialysis in 2009.

So from Grady they crossed the Decatur Street bridge that spans the always-busy I-75/85 Atlanta "downtown connector." They had seen the Mercy Care clinic, near the Reverend Martin Luther King transit station, and thought that maybe the nonprofit, charitable clinic might take him. The intake people at the clinic were helpful, Christina said, but Mercy Care wasn't equipped to provide dialysis.

On their way back to the subway, they also walked past a

for-profit dialysis center. They didn't go inside. The Mercy Care folks had already warned them the for-profit center doesn't take walk-in charity cases.

It seems certain that Eduardo will wind up at Grady. It may take another week or so, but unless he finds a center that will provide the service for free, he is destined to need the Grady ER when his kidneys fail.

This is how one of the nation's most costly, and one of its most unusual health care programs—designed to make kidney dialysis available to anyone who needs it—works. Or, more correctly, in Eduardo Agatone's case, how it leaves thousands of people behind.

Medical science has attempted to replicate failing human organs with machines for decades, but it has only been truly successful at one—the kidney.

Machines that can filter the blood of toxins and other impurities that wreak havoc on the body, a process known as hemodialysis, have been around since the 1940s. But the early versions—they literally were washing-machine-sized tubs next to the patient's bed—often proved more risky than the disease itself.

Even when later improvements in the mechanics and filtration process significantly reduced the risks, dialysis was mostly touted as a stopgap measure for people in the final stages of kidney disease who were awaiting a donor organ for transplant, considered the most ideal treatment for the condition. (Interestingly, this "bridge to transplant" concept is still the primary reason heart failure patients, such as former Vice President Dick Cheney, get artificial hearts and ventricular assist devices implanted today. There is no viable, long-term mechanical replacement for the human heart. Not yet, anyway.)

The success of dialysis in preventing loss of life for people in the last stages of severe kidney disease roughly coincided with the first years of the nation's Medicare program, which was created to provide health care coverage for Americans over the age of sixty-five. This is important, because unlike other chronic and more prevalent conditions such as heart disease, diabetes, and cancer, to name a few, in 1972, kidney disease would get its own special program under Medicare, regardless of the age of the patient afflicted by it.

From the start, the new program was aimed almost exclusively at covering the cost of treatment of the chronic disease. The concept of prevention—helping at-risk patients keep control of their blood sugar levels, blood pressure, and other conditions that bring on kidney problems—was almost an afterthought.

As Medicare did for hospital reimbursement, the new End Stage Renal Disease (ESRD) program created a windfall for the eventual development of dialysis centers nationwide, providing them a fee-for-service payment for costs, plus a profit, for the patients they treated.

The consequences of carving out coverage for this one condition would reverberate for decades to come. Nationwide, its costs would force a rethinking of the wisdom of weighting payment toward treatment instead of prevention.

But in Atlanta, the problems were more practical, and the gaps in the national program provided no help for Grady.

In 2009 the Atlanta hospital was struggling to get back to solvency after years of operating multimillion-dollar deficits. A new governance structure had been created for Grady, removing day-to-day control of the hospital from the political and patronage control of the Fulton-DeKalb Hospital Authority and vesting it instead in a nonprofit corporation of business and community leaders who vowed to turn the aging institution around as quickly as possible.

A big drain on the hospital's bottom line was the outpatient dialysis clinic, which had unreimbursed expenses of $3.5 million to $4 million for patients each year. The vast majority of patients in the clinic were being cared for, even though they had no insurance and did not qualify for Medicaid or Medicare's ESRD program.

Additionally, the equipment in the clinic was old and needed to be replaced in order to meet higher standards to prevent infection and reduce the risk of anemia. Stressing that Grady simply could not continue to absorb such losses, the hospital announced it was closing the outpatient clinic and that its patients would be referred elsewhere.

Of course, it wasn't that simple.

About sixty of the eighty-eight patients the hospital routinely provided dialysis to were immigrants in the country illegally. As a matter of law, these patients did not qualify for coverage under the ESRD program that provided dialysis payment for Americans, regardless of age.

Grady felt obligated to find another provider to take them.

The largest kidney dialysis companies in the world, DaVita Healthcare Partners and Fresenius Medical Care, have dozens of clinics around Atlanta—two of them within blocks of Grady—but they were under no obligation to accept the immigrant patients who could have used their help. What was happening at Grady was not their problem, company spokespeople said. They'd be willing to take some of the patients, but only with at least some compensation for their service.

And then there was this additional bit of irony in Grady's dilemma.

Under federal law, hospitals must treat patients who show up in their emergency rooms with life-threatening conditions, regardless of ability to pay or citizenship status. Without routine dialysis, often two to three times a week, end-stage kidney disease patients can go into full kidney failure within two weeks. They show up in hospital ERs short of breath, confused, and with rapid heart rates. They experience seizures or go into a coma.

When patients present at Grady's ER with these obvious symptoms, they are admitted and stay a few days, getting their dialysis on an inpatient basis, until they are ready for discharge. But after the outpatient dialysis clinic closed in 2009, some of them simply started recycling through the ER and the hospital's inpatient wards, running up other bills that went unpaid.

At this point you might think that state or local governments might step in to help.

You'd be wrong.

Uninsured and Undocumented, a Lethal Combination

At the height of the economic recession, the Fulton and DeKalb county commissions—the two governing bodies directly responsible for Grady's existence—were both reeling from plummeting home values that crippled their local tax base. In the contentious run-up to turning over the hospital's management to a nonprofit corporation, their political appointees to the Fulton-DeKalb Hospital Authority no longer had much clout. So neither county commission was in the mood to increase appropriations for Grady, regardless of the dialysis crisis. The new board would have to deal with this.

State government was even less help.

Georgia's legislature had just gone through several sessions enacting laws largely aimed at making it uncomfortable for illegal immigrants to stay in the state. They tried everything from imposing restrictions on the services county health departments can provide them, to making it easier for local police to arrest and detain traffic violators thought to be in the country illegally.

About this same time, a state university student who had been ticketed for a traffic violation in her campus parking lot was hauled into the Cobb County jail and turned over to federal authorities for failure to show she was in the country legally. When the Feds released her, county authorities filed an additional charge against her alleging she had given them a false address.

That was the climate surrounding illegal immigration in Georgia while Grady was facing a decision about how to manage undocumented people who needed kidney dialysis to stay alive. This, mind you, from a state and metro region whose construction, landscaping, roofing, agriculture, and domestic services industries rely heavily on the hard, cheap labor that undocumented immigrants provide.

Eventually, the hospital came up with a plan.

The undocumented immigrants who were relying on Grady could choose from two options. They could stay in Atlanta and get treatment at one of the commercial dialysis clinics that agreed to accept some of the patients as long as Grady paid for their care. Or the hospital would pay their airfare back to their home countries as well as provide them some cash payments and assistance in finding insurance and dialysis service when they got there.

(The hospital even hired a California company to help its patients repatriate and find medical care back home. The company was paid $18,000 for each patient it assisted, according to a *New York Times* article on the situation.)

The free-trip-home option didn't appeal to many of the patients who not only had families and worked in Atlanta, but who knew enough about their former countries to conclude they would be better off staying in Georgia, even if there was no guarantee they would get the routine dialysis treatments they needed.

Remember too that emergency dialysis always remained an option—not a great option but perhaps better than what they could get at home. They could go to any hospital on an emergency basis. And from a financial perspective, they asked, why return home and earn $10 to $15 a day as a farmhand when they could earn $10 to $12 an hour in Georgia doing roof work or landscaping?

What happened to this handful of immigrants once they left Grady's care is largely unknown.

Most apparently got their care from commercial dialysis centers as long as Grady footed the bill. After that money ran out, some got help from religious groups and local charities to continue their treatment.

But as is often the case with the poor and uninsured in America, most simply disappeared into the health care system, relying on free care where they could get it and indirectly driving up the cost of care for everyone else. Some left for other parts of the country where they could find work and where hostility toward providing them care was not as acute as it was in Georgia. Others, it seems reasonable to surmise, may have died. (Without dialysis or a transplant, end-stage kidney disease is uniformly fatal.)

The *New York Times* followed several of the Grady patients back home in Mexico where their ability to find dialysis as often as they needed was inconsistent, at best. Two of the former patients died, although it is unclear whether their deaths were the result of insufficient dialysis or because their disease had progressed so far that dialysis no longer worked. The father of one of those told the *Times* that his daughter could only afford two dialysis treatments per week in Mexico, compared to the three a week she was getting at Grady before she was forced to leave.

Mexico has no equivalent of Medicare's ESRD program. Those without insurance or the ability to pay for it on their own often die for lack of care, nephrology physicians in Mexico say. They quickly add that they wish their country would adopt a program similar to that in the United States for patients with severe kidney disease.

But the ESRD program in this country has issues of its own that are emblematic of America's fractured and often contradictory approach toward health care for the poor. Although there is little doubt that expanding the program to the hundreds of thousands of Americans who could benefit from it saves lives, it has done so at extraordinary cost. And it remains the only chronic disease that gets singled out for coverage, regardless of income or age status.

Enrolling hundreds of thousands of new patients into the new Medicare program sparked a surge in the private dialysis clinics in the 1980s and 1990s not unlike what happened in the 1960s and 1970s, when private and for-profit hospitals welcomed a whole new market of fully covered elderly patients.

Private investors and publicly traded companies started buying out dialysis clinics that were owned by local nephrologists. They built and purchased dozens of street-corner locations for their clinics in large cities and metro areas with a virtual guarantee of healthy profits. Eventually two companies, Denver-based DaVita Healthcare Partners and Fresenius Medical Care, a German company, took control of 70 percent of the dialysis market in the United States.

Free enterprise at work, right?

Well, *socialized* free enterprise, perhaps, with a hefty dose of financial underpinning by a federal health care program that was originally designed to be available only to the elderly.

Medicare Gets an Unusual Expansion

The bottom-line math of the ESRD program is this: Medicare spends more than $28-$30 billion annually on kidney dialysis and transplantation. About 17,000 patients a year get a donor kidney, the best treatment alternative for the end stage of the disease. But transplantation is limited to the availability of donor organs.

And some kidney disease patients may not even be aware of the transplant option.

A 2015 study by Emory University showed that only about one in four Georgians with kidney disease in their first year of dialysis are referred to transplant centers to be considered for surgery. The study also showed that the dialysis centers with the lowest referral rates were more likely to treat low-income patients who live in poor neighborhoods. Lack of social workers at the dialysis centers may have contributed to the low referral rate, the researchers said.

The shortage of organs and inconsistent referrals for transplantation means about 500,000 patients in the United States must rely on dialysis.

The cost for caring for these patients—who make up just 1 percent of Medicare's total enrollment base of 50 million—is extraordinarily high. They account for about 7 percent of Medicare expenditures each year. Viewed from another perspective, in a given year Medicare spends on average $75,000 on an ESRD patient, compared to about $11,000 for an elderly patient without the disease.

Not surprisingly, as the population has aged, and as precursors to kidney failure such as diabetes and hypertension became more prevalent, government policy makers have tried to rein in the cost of the program.

Their first move, about a decade after the program began, was to set a flat rate of payment for each dialysis session. Then, as new anemia-reduction drugs called erythropoietin-stimulating agents (ESAs) came on the market, Medicare allowed those to be paid for on a fee-for-service basis.

The practical effect was dialysis providers may not have made much on the treatment itself, but they could still make a lot of money on the drugs patients were now routinely getting. Not unexpectedly, the use of ESAs skyrocketed, as did Medicare's overall costs. (In 2014 alone, these protein-based drugs represented $2 billion in Medicare spending.)

It wasn't until 2011 that Medicare decided to "bundle" payment for dialysis services for ESRD program patients by providing a flat fee for treatment, drugs, and testing. That move—and another, yet to be fully implemented, that pays providers based on how well they control dialysis needs and anemia in patients—changed the dynamic in the marketplace. Profitability in dialysis treatment now is centered on higher reimbursement rates the companies get from privately insured patients rather than from ESRD patients. It's little wonder, then, that the for-profit centers eschew charity patients.

Which again brings us back to Grady.

Closing the outpatient dialysis clinic didn't just displace undocumented immigrants in need of care. There were a couple of dozen US citizens without health insurance who used the clinic each week too. They were caught in the gap between the time it takes to get officially designated as suffering from end-stage renal disease and qualifying for the Medicare program.

Americans covered by private insurance, or by insurance they pay for at work, must wait for about a year after diagnosis before qualifying for the Medicare program. These are the most sought-after patients at the for-profit clinics. After a year, most move seamlessly into the ESRD program.

Poor people without insurance have a waiting period too before getting in the ESRD program, usually about three months. But the process can take longer. Some nonprofit clinics take these patients and absorb the cost of dialysis until they qualify for the Medicare program, but many won't accept new patients unless they have a payment source.

A few states have emergency provisions in their Medicaid programs to pay for dialysis for these patients while they wait to qualify. Georgia is one of them, but it discontinued emergency Medicaid coverage for undocumented immigrants in 2006. For poor and undocumented immigrants in the Atlanta area, Grady filled the gap, at a cost of about $6,000 per month per patient, which was what prompted the crisis that forced the closing of the outpatient clinic.

The ESRD program remains the largest federal health initiative designed to provide a medically necessary procedure for people regardless of age or income. There is no other program quite like it in terms of cost and access. Yet it too has significant gaps that the marketplace either cannot, or does not want to, handle. Grady continues to help the people caught in these gaps by referring them to nonprofit centers who might be able to taken them.

Making Progress on Cancer

Dr. Sheryl Gabram is a veteran in the battle to reduce the treatment gap between white and African-American cancer patients.

Dr. Gabram and a specialized team working at the Georgia Cancer Center for Excellence at Grady have their work cut out for them. More than 80 percent of their patients are African-American. Many are poor and have no insurance. At least those over sixty-five have Medicare.

Still, the progress the Grady team is making provides hope that racial disparities in diagnosing and successfully treating chronic diseases such as cancers of the breast, uterus, and colon can be overcome.

Although she is a respected researcher, it didn't take a detailed scientific study for Dr. Gabram to determine one of the most significant predictors of treatment success.

As a breast cancer surgeon affiliated with both Grady and Emory University's Winship Cancer Institute, Dr. Gabram is often the first physician to sit down with patients to tell them they have cancer. She goes over in some detail the results of their biopsies, imaging, and other tests so they can start making decisions about how aggressive their treatment should be.

Not surprisingly, the patients at Winship are predominantly white and are covered by Medicare or private insurance. When she sees patients at Winship, Dr. Gabram said, almost all of them are with a loved one—most often a spouse, but sometimes a child, a sibling, or a close friend—when they get the news. But when she meets with her patients at Grady to tell them about their cancer, 95 percent of them are alone.

Years of research have shown that breast cancer patients who have family or friends at their side while they go through surgery, chemotherapy, radiation, and long-term hormonal therapy uniformly do better and finish their treatment. Patients who have no support are more likely to put off treatment, or skip it altogether.

Even after successful surgery to remove cancerous tumors, skipping their follow-up care greatly increases the risk that the cancer will return. This failure to get the full treatment they need is one of the reasons poor, black patients fare worse than whites—both in recurrence and in mortality.

But the primary reason for poorer outcomes is that black women are less likely to be screened for breast cancer in the first place. Many black women are unaware of their family's medical history, are less likely to have a primary care physician, and are more likely to be uninsured or have inadequate insurance coverage that would pay for a mammogram.

A large study of patients in the fifty most populous US cities puts the challenge into perspective.

While the overall mortality rate for breast cancer between 1990 and 2009 declined, the decrease among black women was much slower, only about half of what it was among whites. In fact, in thirty-five cities the disparity in mortality actually widened.

The study, paid for by the Avon Foundation for Women, was the first to put a number to the death toll: 1,710 African-American women die each year (that works out to five a day) due to racial disparities in screening and breast cancer treatment.

The findings didn't surprise Dr. Gabram, whose Grady breast cancer center has received about $20 million in funding from the Avon Foundation over the years.

"It's very, very frustrating that we still see patients with late-stage disease," she said. "We know that we can make a difference if we get to these women early and keep them in treatment, so that's where we have concentrated our resources."

Dr. Gabram and cancer experts at a handful of other public hospitals in urban areas around the country have struck on a solution that seems to work.

Many long-standing programs use breast cancer survivors as community health advocates These are women who are trained to provide information at health fairs, neighborhood meetings, and in school and church settings about the risks of cancer and where to get low-cost or no-cost mammograms. But the Grady team took this concept one step further. They trained twenty of their advocates to become patient navigators to help find and convince at-risk women to be tested, as well as help them during their often-confusing journey through surgery and follow-up treatment.

The navigators work closely with the hospital's social services and nursing staff as well as the clinic's multidisciplinary breast tumor team in understanding the patient's progress at each stage of treatment, so they can translate what comes next.

But at its most simple and effective level, the navigators are there—often by phone, but in home and clinic visits as well—to remind patients when their next chemotherapy session is scheduled, or to ask whether they have had any unusual side effects of chemo or radiation that they want the medical team to know about.

In so doing, the low-income patients who may have started their cancer journey alone come to understand they have someone who is closely monitoring their care. They are more likely to complete their treatment, less likely to have the disease come back, and less likely to die from it.

The results from this approach at the Grady clinic have been encouraging, now that the program has been running for several years, Dr. Gabram said.

In one fifteen-month period, the community health advocates reached 9,600 women and identified hundreds who were at risk for breast cancer and never had a mammogram.

Within a few days of their encounters with at-risk women, Grady's patient navigators were on the phone giving them information about where to get screening mammograms and whether they qualify for special coverage for their tests through the Georgia Cancer Screening Program, a joint CDC–State of Georgia program aimed at early detection of breast and cervical cancer among low-income women in the state.

The Importance of Early Action

The vast majority of these patients would probably have foregone getting a checkup, Dr. Gabram said, and many of them would have eventually shown up with late-stage disease.

Additionally, a goal of the program is to reduce the time it takes from diagnosis of the disease to treatment, which not that long ago at Grady was often six months or more. Again, one persistent disparity between black and white breast cancer patients in the United States is in how much longer black women have to wait to start chemotherapy and other treatments after their surgery.

When Dr. Gabram and other researchers compared treatment times of patients at Grady with a private community hospital in Atlanta from 2004 to 2008, they found that African-American patients at Grady tended to wait longer between having a core biopsy (indicating the presence of cancer) to undergoing surgery to remove the tumor and getting a definitive pathological staging of the disease. Staging the disease as precisely as possible is important for making decisions about postsurgical treatment, including chemotherapy and radiation, to prevent recurrence of the disease.

What causes the delay toward treatment among black women was difficult to pinpoint. But there were some predictors. Unmarried women were more likely to wait longer.

Lack of transportation to get to appointments also tended to cause delays.

Once again, patient navigators and better-coordinated care could make a big difference, Dr. Gabram concluded.

By concentrating resources on the community outreach level—one of the goals of the Avon Foundation–sponsored program—the Grady advocates and navigators have begun to reduce the gap between the races in Atlanta. Other urban hospitals around the country are employing similar approaches.

But Dr. Gabram and her team do not stop there. The Grady specialists are committed to providing the highest standard of care for breast cancer patients who might not otherwise be able to afford it.

The multidisciplinary team at Grady works closely with experts at Emory's Winship Cancer Institute, the only NCI-designated comprehensive cancer center in Georgia. The women diagnosed with late-stage disease at Grady have their cases reviewed by the team and are also enrolled, whenever possible, in clinical trials for new cancer drugs and targeted treatment protocols.

Moreover, the Grady program was quick to find resources to make a huge advancement in breast cancer care—tumor profiling—available to their low-income patients.

Tumor profiling, also known as gene expression profiling, provides women in early stages of breast cancer more information about their treatment options. Knowing the specific genetic composition of the cancer cells helps clinicians determine more precisely how useful chemotherapy can be, or whether it could be skipped altogether.

But gene-profiling tests are not cheap. They often range between $3,000 and $5,000. Insurance coverage is not always guaranteed, which has traditionally been a stumbling block in rolling out expensive new medical modalities.

Prior to this important development, women in the early stages of the disease—even those whose cancer had not spread to nearby lymph nodes—almost always got several rounds of chemotherapy to guard against a recurrence of the disease. Gene profiling is very predictive of the chances for recurrence of the disease, and women with a low genetic risk can make a more informed decision about whether to undergo the endurance trial that months of chemotherapy entails.

Moving so quickly to make scientific and clinical advances available to low-income cancer patients like those at Grady is unusual in our health care system. Numerous studies have shown that new technologies and procedures in American medicine are made available to affluent and well-insured patients years before they are deployed for poor and uninsured patients. This is another reason why disparities in outcomes between white and black patients exist for chronic diseases, such as cancer.

An April 2015 study in the respected policy journal *Health Affairs* showed there was a wide gap in the use of gene expression profiling within communities where there is significant income inequality. Insured patients with the highest income were more likely to be offered—and to take advantage of—gene expression testing than lower-income patients, even those with insurance. That's not too surprising since many insured patients may not be able to shell out $4,000 of their own for the test if their insurance doesn't cover it.

But, viewed from a different perspective, it is also short-sighted on the insurer's part. If a $4,000 test finds that half of a company's enrollees asking for it can forgo chemotherapy, the insurer stands to save millions in potentially unnecessary treatment costs.

(The costs of chemotherapy drugs alone often run $20,000 to $40,000. Drugs to deal with the side effects and to regenerate infection-fighting white blood cells depressed from chemotherapy often run several thousand dollars more.)

The *Health Affairs* study was the first to demonstrate an association with income inequality in a community, not just that low-income patients are often left behind when it comes to technological advances in treatment. The greater the inequality of income in the marketplace, the researchers found, the more likely only the affluent would get the test.

The study holds particular significance now because many of the insurance policies available under the ACA exchanges carry high deductibles and are restrictive when it comes to covering emerging technologies such as gene profiling.

All the more reason, Dr. Gabram said, why Grady's program must search for independent funding sources and other ways to get poor and low-income women the quality of care other American women take for granted.

But public policy must acknowledge and deal with the gaps as well, said Dr. Otis W. Brawley, the chief medical officer of the American Cancer Society and Dr. Gabram's predecessor at the Georgia Cancer Center for Excellence at Grady.

"We must own up to the fact that these disparities exist and deal with them at every level: access to insurance, access to care, access to quality care," Dr. Brawley said.

Groups like the Cancer Society, the Avon Foundation, Susan G. Komen, and others can raise awareness and provide some funding for initiatives like the Grady center, but until the country develops a health care system that is fair and equitable to all Americans, it will be an uphill battle.

For now, it seems evident that the nation's public hospitals will have to staff the front lines of that battle to reduce racial and income disparities in the treatment of chronic conditions.

And they will need to do it while remaining the first, and most important, institutions in many communities to provide essential and costly services for other serious conditions that most of their competitors would like to avoid.

8

ON THE FRONT LINES OF AIDS, FUNDING REMAINS UNCERTAIN

Having moved to Atlanta when he was in middle school, Jonathan quickly discovered the city could be a haven for young black men who were protective of their sexual identity.

In Atlanta, he said, he wasn't scorned or picked on because he was gay, not even during those always-tough high school years. He loved the city. He was comfortable there.

Still, he never expected his aunt would kick him out of her apartment where he was living at the time when she learned he was gay. When that happened, everything changed.

After graduating from high school, he worked a series of part-time jobs, sharing rooms with friends. He was careful, he said, about sex with friends and strangers.

Jonathan came of age during a time when HIV was "just another illness—we all know it's out there," he said. But he readily admits now that he wasn't careful enough.

When he was diagnosed with HIV in late 2012 at eighteen years of age, he said, "It didn't surprise me, I guess. It's just unbelievable because you never think it will happen to you."

Whether Jonathan's actions speak to his youthful naiveté or the willful ignorance of a new generation of sexually active gay and bisexual men doesn't much matter to the staff of Grady Hospital's Infectious Disease Program. The staff at the hospital's IDP has been taking care of HIV patients for over two decades. Its patient rolls now top more than five thousand. It is one of a handful of comprehensive HIV clinics in the nation, almost all of them affiliated with large urban hospitals that continue to form the nation's front line against the epidemic.

In recent years, Grady clinic administrators say, the rise in the number of HIV-positive patients between the ages of thirteen and twenty-four has become a major concern, not just in Atlanta but in almost all the major cities in the South. While clinical medicine has made great strides in the treatment of HIV—so much so that the condition is no longer considered the death sentence it once was—the cost for such care can be staggeringly high.

The cocktail of drugs needed to keep the virus in check can cost a thousand dollars or more per month. But public health experts believe the cost is more than offset if the viral loads of HIV-positive men are kept so low they can stay healthy and reduce the chances of spreading the disease to their sex partners.

How AIDS clinics like the one at Grady are financed in the future is a major public health issue that has yet to be adequately addressed. The 2010 Affordable Care Act was supposed to deal with it, but because states don't have to expand Medicaid coverage—as the act envisioned they would—poor, uninsured HIV patients, like Jonathan, and the hospitals that care for them, could lose access to the treatment they need to stay well and keep from spreading the disease.

Moreover, the future of the federal program used for two decades to help provide services to poor HIV-infected patients is caught up in the acrimonious debate in Washington over health care financing.

All this uncertainty is deepening as the epidemic has taken an alarming turn.

In just one day in 2013, the Grady program treated seventeen new teenage HIV cases, according to Jacqueline T. Muther, the former HIV policy, contracts, and resource manager for the Atlanta clinic. This was the year the clinic felt the true impact of the new trend line, which has continued in more recent years but not with the alarming numbers seen in 2013.

Seventeen new patients in one day wouldn't otherwise be a

big deal at the Grady clinic, one of the largest in the Southeast. But these seventeen had much in common.

"All of them were young. All of them were sick." And many of them had only recently been tested for the first time, before being referred to the Grady clinic, she recalled. "It was like we were starting this whole epidemic over again. When that happens, it gets your attention."

Many of the new patients fit Jonathan's profile. (Jonathan is not his real name. He chose it to protect his identity because some of his family members are still unaware of his health status.) After moving out of his aunt's house, he went several times for free HIV testing using a swab of saliva from his mouth, always to find out he was negative for the virus. Perhaps that made him feel immune to the need for extra caution, he said.

But then he started feeling sick all the time and began losing weight. Uninsured, he went to a Grady internal medicine clinic where doctors ordered a complete blood profile. "I had been tired for so long, and I was just tired of being afraid. I knew something was wrong," he said about the day he finally went to the clinic. "It was like I was already dying."

The following day, two workers from Grady's IDP showed up at his door. The tests showed the virus was wearing out his immune system's ability to deal with it. He went with them immediately to the specialized clinic to start a regimen of drugs and enroll in counseling and social service programs. Within four months, the virus was under control, and Jonathan's life had stabilized.

New Concerns about Where the Epidemic Is Heading

This disconcerting change in the trajectory of the epidemic raises huge issues, and not unlike in the early years of AIDS in America, no one is sure how it will play out.

During the 1990s, there was some hope of reaching a peak in the epidemic as the overall rate of new infections began to decline. But the success was never shared equally within demographic groups of the at-risk population. The rate for HIV remains stubbornly higher among African-Americans than whites.

But what has the attention of HIV experts now is that between 2001 and 2011, the annual diagnoses of HIV among gay and bisexual men ages thirteen to twenty-four of all races more than doubled, compared to the decade before that.

(Epidemiologists like to analyze trend lines over five- to ten-year spans. This trend of new infections among young men stood out as one of the most important in the first decade of the 2000s. From more recent surveillance data, the proportion of cases among adolescents and young adults has held steady in the second decade as well, experts say.)

In 2010 alone, 25 percent of all new infections in the United States were among thirteen-to-twenty-four-year-old gay and bisexual men. The most likely reason for the spike? Ignorance and risky behavior by a new generation of men who don't fear AIDS like their predecessors did.

Moreover, this age group is much more likely to use injection drugs and much less likely to be voluntarily tested for HIV. For them, the stigma of homosexuality remains very real, experts say, but the fear of AIDS doesn't.

A 2014 study by Emory University epidemiologists showed that gay and bisexual black men in Atlanta have a 60 percent chance of becoming infected with HIV by the age of thirty. Overall, the rate of black males living with HIV in Atlanta is more than four times what it is for white men.

The reasons for the disparity are complicated, but research seems to indicate that gay and bisexual black men are more likely to have sex with black men than they are with white men, compounding the percentage of infected persons since the rate among black men is higher to start with.

Moreover, white gay and bisexual men are much more

likely than their black counterparts to have health insurance and access to medications that help control HIV, thus reducing the risk of transmission to their sex partners.

National surveys of large cities show similar patterns, although not quite as alarming as the 2014 findings about Atlanta. Still, the rate of new infections in the urban core of America's largest cities—especially those in the South—also corresponds to areas of the country where adult males are likely to be poor and unemployed and have no health insurance.

These observations help explain why new cases are disproportionately coming in the Southern states and their big cities, like Atlanta, Miami, Houston, and New Orleans.

The CDC first reported this trend line of new cases in 2010. More specifically, new infections in Texas, Louisiana, Mississippi, Alabama, Tennessee, Georgia, Florida, and South Carolina seemed to be driving the high rates for the entire region. (These eight states had a new diagnosis rate of 23.8 per 100,000 residents, more than twice the rate of the Midwestern states and significantly higher than any other region.)

That same year, nine of the ten metropolitan regions nationwide with the highest HIV diagnosis rates were in these states.

It's uncertain whether the outsized role that Southern states have played since the epidemic reached its third decade has continued, but it seems likely. The Grady clinic continues to see a high number of new cases among 15-24-year-old males, Muther said, sometimes as many as 20 a day. The demand has been so high that the clinic sets aside one day of the week to ensure newly enrolled patients sign up for the services they need.

A June 2015 report from the CDC shows the extent of the challenge. Texas, Florida, and Georgia account for three of the top five states nationwide thought to have the largest number of undiagnosed HIV cases in the country. Louisiana showed up as number ten.

This is important because another survey released by the Kaiser Family Foundation in 2014 showed fewer than 20 percent of gay and bisexual men have been tested for HIV in the last six months, and almost one in three have never been tested. Anecdotally, many providers note, teenagers and young adults are even less likely to be regularly tested.

"We also know that these patients are the hardest to keep on track because they move around a lot," Muther of the Grady clinic said. "They get sick, get tested, and learn their status for the first time, and then they disappear. It's quite discouraging because we know that with continuity of care we can help them."

Something has gone badly wrong. With the benefit of nearly thirty years of research that has produced better drugs and advanced treatment protocols, these young patients should not be facing the bleak outcome the first AIDS patients did. There are more than 1.1 million Americans with HIV alive today. They are living with a condition that once caused death within a year or two of diagnosis.

And with the Affordable Care Act and its prohibition against denying individual health insurance coverage for people with chronic conditions, the newest generation of patients should also be able to afford to manage their disease, or at least that was the conventional wisdom at the time the law was passed in 2010.

Unfortunately, the hoped-for results from the ACA have yet to materialize for many HIV/AIDS patients.

Underinsured in a New Era of High-Cost Drugs

Advocates in Georgia, Illinois, Florida, and elsewhere have noted many of those who gained coverage for the first time are saddled with plans that inadequately cover the drugs they need, if they cover them at all. Others face huge deductibles that they hadn't really counted on paying.

During the first full year of the ACA, after hearing from

hundreds of patients facing these and other issues, the non-profit AIDS Institute filed a formal complaint with the federal government over how four insurance companies selling policies on the Florida ACA exchange structured their drug coverage and benefits.

Carl Schmid, deputy executive director of the institute, believed the insurance companies were pricing their individual plans with high out-of-pocket spending purposely to keep HIV patients from enrolling.

Illinois advocates said they heard similar concerns about lack of drug coverage and high costs from HIV patients now covered under the ACA.

"We're seeing a variety of problems for a lot of patients who have out-of-network providers or medications that aren't in the provider's formulary," said Kathye Gorosh, senior vice president of the AIDS Foundation of Chicago. "There is a lot of uncertainty. We're still very concerned about access and costs."

The problem was serious enough that the Illinois Department of Insurance, which supervises the state's individual policy exchange under the ACA, warned insurance companies in 2014 that failure to cover the ACA's list of "preferred" or "alternative" HIV drug regimens in the plans they sell could be considered an act of discrimination.

The health insurance industry denies companies are purposely writing policies to screen out HIV enrollees. But insurers have heard the concerns and will be adjusting details of the plans they offer in the years to come, according to its leading trade group.

Escalating drug costs—for many diseases, not just HIV—will always impact policy premiums and out-of-pocket expenses, the industry said. Under the new law, consumers are given the option of choosing higher-cost premiums in exchange for having to pay less out of their own pockets for drugs.

The "tiered" system created by the ACA allows insurance companies to charge a greater share to the patient for the cost of newer, expensive drugs, while keeping out-of-pocket charges to a bare minimum—sometimes at no patient cost at all—for older, generic drugs in the least-expensive tier.

That's the good news/bad news element of the ACA. For the first time, thanks to the new law, HIV patients can't be banned from getting coverage. But even with insurance, they may not be able to afford the treatment they need, especially if they opt for a policy with low-cost premiums that forces them to pay more for the drugs they use.

Gorosh and other advocates acknowledge that there is a steep learning curve for HIV patients new to the individual insurance market when it comes to understanding how insurance networks and their drug formularies operate. In the first round of enrollment under the new law, many patients were simply looking for the plan with the cheapest monthly premium and didn't understand their drug benefit, she believes.

That can be a challenge for HIV/AIDS patients and others with chronic conditions who are taking multiple medications daily. Most importantly, continued success at fighting the disease and keeping it from spreading to others is directly related to strict compliance with the prescribed drug regimens.

The stakes are high, not just for the patients who might risk getting sick because they can't afford their medications, but for the providers who have to find a way to absorb the costs if the patients can't pay out of their own pockets. Many of the plans require patients to put up half the cost of the expensive drugs they need, a tab that can easily run up to $1,000 a month for HIV patients. (There is a cap on out-of-pocket expenses of about $6,200 per year per patient under most plans sold through the exchanges.)

Newer, more effective drugs and drug combinations for HIV and other infectious diseases are always expensive when they first come on the market. That's not likely to change anytime soon, and it will continue to impact the cost of insurance coverage.

For instance, relatively recent, but highly effective drugs

for hepatitis C—a chronic liver disease impacting 3.2 million Americans, and one that kills about 15,000 people a year—costs $84,000 to $95,000 for a twelve-week course of treatment. The drug Sovaldi is considered a major breakthrough in the disease because it has the ability to cure patients and is much less toxic than the conventional drugs that have been prescribed in the past to manage the condition. (About one in five patients at the Grady clinic is also infected with hepatitis C.)

Because of the cost, Medicaid officials in several states have announced they are considering some kind of limit on which Medicaid patients get the expensive drugs and when. Oregon, for instance, said the new drug would cost the state $360 million in 2014 for Medicaid patients who qualified. That's only $17 million less than the state program has budgeted for the same year on all prescription drugs for its 600,000 Medicaid recipients.

The Oregon approach requires Medicaid patients to have advanced liver disease before they even qualify to get the drugs. Plus, they must agree not to drink alcohol or use illicit drugs for at least a year before treatment.

But at least Oregon has decided to expand Medicaid to cover more of the working poor who did not qualify for the federal-state program in the past.

The Medicaid Gap and Ryan White Funding

Many states—including most Southern states—have elected not to extend Medicaid coverage under the ACA to thousands of poor and low-income HIV/AIDS patients. In these states, current Medicaid enrollment is largely limited to pregnant woman, their newborn babies, and the elderly disabled. Most able-bodied adults under age sixty-five don't qualify, but many don't make enough money to afford private insurance, even with the federal subsidies that are provided.

At the Grady clinic in Atlanta, about 80 percent of the patients are African-American and 60 percent live below the federal poverty level. Had Georgia decided to expand Medicaid, clinic administrators estimate that about half of the uninsured patients they treat would have qualified.

Even in those states that have embraced the ACA, some vital services for successful treatment of HIV/AIDS patients—case management, social support, and housing—are not covered by the state Medicaid program or private insurers selling plans on the state exchange.

Confounding all this is the future of the Ryan White Act, a two-decade-old federal program considered "the payer of last resort" for poor and uninsured Americans with HIV.

The act is supposed to be covering at least some of the uninsured patients left behind in the states that refuse to expand Medicaid, but deciding which patients and what services are covered has been difficult, at best, clinic administrators say. That makes budgeting almost impossible, and to a person, all of them worry that funding for the program in the future could get caught up in the partisan rancor within Congress over the ACA and other health care legislation.

In 2014 the Ryan White Act spent more than $2.3 billion on HIV/AIDS education, prevention, and treatment programs. But funding for it is "discretionary," meaning it is not an entitlement program like Medicare and must be authorized each year by Congress. Since the passage of the ACA, yearly funding for the Ryan White program has remained essentially flat.

Moreover, had Medicaid expansion been enacted nationwide, Ryan White funding could have been shifted toward education, prevention, and social service efforts while Medicaid picked up the cost of treatment. Without it, those programs must continue to compete against each other in non-Medicaid expansion states.

That's not encouraging news for HIV programs at hospitals

like Grady that form the public health infrastructure for treating poor and uninsured patients with HIV, hepatitis, and other sexually transmitted diseases.

Public Hospitals Filling the Gaps

Since the early days of the AIDS epidemic, infectious disease experts, medical social workers, epidemiologists, and other specialists working at these clinics have constituted the front lines of clinical care—taking on the challenge when colleagues in private practice were too cautious, or unwilling, to accept infected patients.

San Francisco General Hospital was among the first to create a comprehensive line of services for hundreds of HIV/AIDS patients when most other communities were still months and years away from encountering their first patients infected by the virus.

The hospital opened a dedicated inpatient unit in 1983 about the same time it created an outpatient clinic that became home to thousands of gay, middle-class men who otherwise would have sought care using private-practice physicians and at private community hospitals. The services provided at San Francisco General became a model for other large, urban hospitals in the years to come.

Still, these hospitals had to adapt their services to the specific needs of the communities they served.

New York City, another site where hundreds of cases first were identified, had a complex combination of HIV-infected men and women seeking care in its public hospitals. Besides the middle-class, gay white men from Greenwich Village who showed up needing care, North Central Bronx Hospital also had to deal with injection-drug users who were infected by using contaminated needles, as well as their heterosexual partners.

This cross section of patients forced public health providers to address issues of drug abuse and prostitution, among other things, besides educating the at-risk population about the virus itself.

The HIV/AIDS story was altogether different in Miami and South Florida.

Jackson Memorial Hospital, like other major urban hospitals in the early days of the epidemic, had its share of gay men being treated for HIV. But it faced a much more difficult challenge among the Haitian community, which was not just poor but marginalized within Miami's rich ethnic diversity. Whereas HIV patients in San Francisco, New York, Los Angeles, and other large cities were dying most often from cancer, the poor Haitian immigrants infected with HIV in Miami died overwhelmingly and quickly from pneumonia and toxoplasmosis, a common parasitic infection.

Pathologists at Jackson Memorial were among the first to identify how pregnant women infected with the virus could pass it to their unborn babies—a finding that eventually led to a prenatal protocol for treating infected women that has effectively ended mother-to-child transmission during childbirth.

The HIV experience at Chicago's John H. Stroger, Jr. Hospital of Cook County is more typical of how most urban public hospitals deal with the epidemic today.

Dr. Mardge Cohen, director of HIV research at the Ruth M. Rothstein CORE Center, an affiliate of the county hospital, recalled how doctors and nurses were pressed into service in the first years of the epidemic to treat the hospital's predominantly working poor and minority patients. "The people who took on the care of these patients saw it as a mission, a passion. If not us, who would do this?" she said.

The forerunner of the CORE center opened in 1983 and quickly saw what other urban providers were also encountering—women with AIDS. The Chicago clinic assembled a team of HIV specialists who created a family-centered program for women and children, one that emphasized mental health, substance abuse, and housing services.

The success of many of these urban HIV clinics is directly linked to community services outside the hospital walls, as well as medical services not traditionally performed by hospital staff. One of the most important services involves oral health care. The Grady clinic was one of the first in the country to recognize this.

One Doctor, One Patient, and a New Mission

Dr. David Reznik was in private dental practice in Atlanta in the mid-1980s when an HIV-positive patient called his office to make an appointment. Even though he advertised and promoted his practice to Atlanta's gay community, the would-be patient was angry and threatening his receptionist, who happened to be Reznik's mother. So he took the call and scheduled the patient for the next day.

"I understood his anger. He had been turned down by dentists all over town and had no place to go," Reznik recalled. "He had dental insurance coverage, but no one would take him."

After a simple dental cleaning for his new patient, Reznik—having learned nothing about HIV while in dental school—bleached all the office equipment he had used, just to be safe.

One HIV patient quickly turned into two, and then a dozen and then a steady stream of Atlanta patients with HIV and AIDS who came to rely on Reznik for their care. During this time he saw a variety of what he called "truly bizarre oral conditions"—cancers, fungal infections, and unusual mouth sores—all associated with HIV.

He started calling dentists and oral health experts at the University of California, San Francisco and in Los Angeles and New York to understand how they were treating HIV patients and to fill them in on what he was seeing. The informal network he helped create eventually became the HIV Dental Alliance (HIVdent), which remains today the go-to source for dental health information in the treatment of HIV patients.

With an HIV patient load of nearly a dozen a day, by 1988 Reznik's work brought him to the attention of Georgia public health officials, Grady Hospital, and AID Atlanta, an advocacy group headed by Sandra Thurmond, who went on to became director of National AIDS Policy under President Clinton.

They asked Reznik to begin taking HIV patients and accept a sliding fee for their care based on their level of income. He did, and when Grady created a comprehensive AIDS treatment program in the city in 1993, Reznik persuaded the hospital to include oral health as part of it.

He's been there ever since, working out of a basement dental office in the Grady Infectious Disease Program clinic that is brightly decorated with dozens of photographs of Diana Ross, his favorite entertainer.

"The mouth is a window to the rest of the body," Reznik said. Oral disease can be the first indication of HIV that patients encounter. Untreated candidiasis, commonly known as thrush, can lead to esophageal candidiasis, an AIDS-defining condition.

Moreover, infections and mouth sores can also be quite painful. To deal with the conditions, some patients resort to drugs, which increases the risk of other unhealthy behaviors.

Upwards of 90 percent of the patients he saw in the early days of the epidemic had severe periodontal disease. "Some of these patients in their twenties or thirties have the gums of what you would normally see in patients in their sixties or seventies," he said. "It's so important for them to get on a treatment plan and get on it quickly."

Over the years, Reznik has become one of Atlanta's most vocal AIDS advocates. The number of patients he's treated who eventually succumbed to the disease, "is too many to count, but I think about all of them, especially in the early years," he said. "The death toll was so high and so discouraging."

He's lost good friends and a partner he loved to the disease. It bothers him sometimes, he said, when he sees young HIV patients who are unaware of the history of the epidemic and how long it took to get to the point that they can expect to live a long time with the proper treatment.

So much has changed, but the young folks he treats now are no less deserving than the first patients who came to him years ago. What bothers him most, he said, is that the success of recent treatments has lulled the public into thinking the epidemic is no longer a major public health threat.

A former member of the National AIDS Advisory Council under President George W. Bush, Reznik vows that he will not allow complacency about AIDS to slow the progress on treatment and prevention of the disease.

"We still are seeing 50,000 new cases a year in this country, and we have yet to come to grips with how to pay for what our patients need," he said. "That means more advocacy work and paying renewed attention to the problem. We've come so far, but we still haven't come to grips with whether everyone should have equal access to quality care. "

9

MENTAL HEALTH: THE CONTINUING CRISIS IN CARING FOR THE POOR

Her psychiatric social worker didn't know why. It could have been lack of money or not having a way to get there, but Juanita's mental stability seemed to hinge on a shopping trip to Target.

"I think she needs some bras," a member of Grady Hospital's Assertive Community Treatment team tells her colleagues as they go through, one by one, a long list of names staring at them on the whiteboard. "It's made her increasingly anxious."

"I'll get you some money," the team's leader said. Another team member jumps in, volunteering to take Juanita to Target the next day.

The next name on the team's board is Peggy, who has temporarily stopped taking her antipsychotic medications, a team member reports. Peggy presented herself at Grady's ER two days before with a urinary tract infection, and she claimed the ER nurses told her that her medications probably caused her infection.

"I had to sit down with her and go over her discharge papers to show her that's not what they were saying," the psychiatric nurse presenting the case tells the team. The next team member who sees her should follow up that she is taking both her psychiatric meds and the antibiotic she was prescribed for her infection.

Two down. The team has about fifty-eight names to go— all patients with similar stories revealing precarious control over their illnesses.

To me, an outside observer who agreed as a condition of attending the meeting not to use the real names of their clients, the team's ability to succeed with many of the patients seems equally precarious, especially given how fragmented and unresponsive the American health care system can be for the chronically mentally ill.

There are success stories, to be certain. The team cheers news of a new job for one of the patients, or a new, more stable living arrangement for another. Robert has reconciled with his brother, who says he'll give him another chance. Rose got her old job back. Jackie's estranged daughter has moved back to town, and she sees her once a week.

But even these patients are one unlucky break away from trouble. Something as random as an argument with a family member, a late Social Security check, an arrest for disorderly conduct, a frustrated municipal court judge who is tired of dealing with them can put them in jeopardy.

The team effort employed at Grady has been around for years. It was first successfully used in Wisconsin and based on a simple, but expensive premise: Chronic, severe mental illness requires more than short-term hospital stays, periodic outpatient group therapy, and daily medications. It involves frequent, supportive contact that ensures patients don't get sidetracked by what most of us would consider minor setbacks, like needing to go shopping. Most importantly, patients must be willing to agree to frequent interventions in order to participate in the program.

Grady has three Assertive Community Treatment teams that meet every weekday. Combined, they have a patient load nearing two hundred—by far the largest of any program like it in Georgia. Funding for the program comes from a variety of sources such as state and local grants, mostly, but also from Medicaid, if the patients are eligible for coverage.

Unfortunately, many aren't. They could be, but Georgia won't allow it. So the program stays permanently underfunded, forcing Grady to absorb the cost.

The goal for each team is to see patients at least three times a week. These encounters are designed to determine if the patients are taking the medications they need, keeping their appointments, having any luck at finding work, and living somewhere that doesn't exacerbate their serious mental conditions.

The Grady program is handling an ever-increasing load because—to put it bluntly—the state of Georgia has failed miserably in stepping up to provide the care these and thousands of patients like them need. And when the state system for caring for the poor and uninsured mentally ill essentially collapses, as it did in Georgia over the last ten years, it predictably falls on public hospitals and nonprofit charities to pick up the pieces.

If there is one medical condition where American medicine and public health policy has failed the poor and uninsured most, it is in mental health care. Despite numerous scandals and journalistic investigations over the years, public officials have rarely put forth efforts to comprehensively deal with it. Think of the last time a political campaign—any political campaign at any level—had a platform promising to fix the obvious failures in mental health financing or services for the poor.

What little progress that has been made on the subject has been to destigmatize chronic depression, bipolar disorders, schizophrenia, addiction, substance abuse, and other conditions as something more than just bad behavior. But "mainstreaming" those disorders has largely been limited to patients who voluntarily submit to treatment and are covered by insurance when they need it.

Underlining the point, in the 1980s and 1990s, as mental health advocates began to make headway in demanding insurance companies cover psychiatric conditions the same way they cover other health issues, there was a surge in for-profit and private psychiatric hospitals opening to accommodate the demand.

Usually covered treatment began with a hospital stay to reestablish a medication regimen, followed by outpatient visits for psychotherapy, counseling, and medication compliance. How long the hospital stay was and how long outpatient care lasted depended largely on what was allowed under the patient's benefit plan. This is still largely the model used today for insured patients who need help coping with their illness.

But for the poor and uninsured, it is a much different world.

Private psychiatric hospitals and some acute-care hospitals with psychiatric beds may accept uninsured patients, often only to stabilize them and discharge them to their own care. But for the most part, these patients become the responsibility of the state mental health system, regional public health districts, the local public hospital, and, increasingly, the local jail and criminal justice system.

"Behavioral health for the poor is one of our most serious challenges, not just from the standpoint of what sworks and what doesn't, but because the numbers are overwhelming, and our system for paying for it has been cobbled together in crisis," said Dr. Bruce Siegel, president and CEO of America's Essential Hospitals, which represents most of the nation's largest safety-net hospitals. "Many states have simply defaulted on public mental health services and expect our hospitals to take on the responsibility."

Moreover, the promise of the 2010 health care reform law to provide coverage for more of the poor and uninsured—either through expanding Medicaid or through private plans that denied them coverage in the past—has also failed to materialize for many of these patients.

About twenty states, including Georgia, have refused to expand Medicaid coverage to residents who make too little to afford private insurance and too much to qualify for Medicaid under current guidelines. That effectively shuts out most of the uninsured mentally ill from the benefits of the new law. And it shifts much of the burden of paying for the care they inevitably need from the state onto public hospitals who have to treat them on an emergency basis.

The American Mental Health Counselors Association estimates that about one million Americans in need of mental health and substance abuse treatment did not receive it in 2014 because their states refused to expand Medicaid to cover them; more than 230,000 of these low-income and vulnerable patients reside in Georgia.

Avoiding Public Responsibility

Over the last fifty years, the states and federal government have attempted to shift the burden of public health funding from one to the other with neither seemingly willing to accept the responsibility for coordinating care for a vulnerable and difficult-to-treat segment of society.

And while there is no winner in this standoff between federal and state health officials, there is no question who is harmed the most. The losers can easily be found on the streets of major cities, in county jails, and in overcrowded public hospital psychiatric wards.

The dismal record spans more than a century of public-policy indifference, stingy funding, unintended consequences, and fundamental misunderstanding of the nature of mental illness itself.

Unlike other chronic health conditions—such as heart disease, kidney disease, or even cancer, where symptoms are easy to diagnose and surgical treatment and medications can mitigate the impact of malfunctioning organs—chronic, serious bipolar disorders and schizophrenia manifest themselves in behavioral patterns that often are not easy to detect and even harder to control.

Insurance companies around the country report that they are having difficulty complying with the requirement written into the 2010 ACA that they treat mental illness on a parity with any other chronic medical condition they cover. They complain that how to best diagnose and treat mental conditions is constantly evolving, making it difficult for insurers, especially HMOs, to provide adequate staff to meet what has turned out to be an unanticipated demand among newly insured patients.

In California, considered the "pace car of parity" for coverage of mental illness, Kaiser Permanente, which insures 7.5 million members in the state, was fined for not providing timely care to mentally ill patients. Its defense was that it did not have the staff and the paperwork requirements in place to monitor compliance with the law. (It does now, the company said.)

While there is no surgical procedure to deal with severe mental illness, fortunately there are drugs to control it. But treatment involves strict compliance and a supportive environment for those afflicted with the most serious forms of these illnesses. For many individuals, especially the poor, the supportive environment simply doesn't exist and must be taken up by the public health system.

Grady CEO John Haupert said the cost of behavioral health services for hundreds of severely mentally ill patients is one of the biggest threats to the bottom line of the state's largest safety-net provider. The high cost of services Grady must provide—especially to those patients who return time and again for inpatient care because they can't take care of themselves—crowds out the hospital's ability to provide care for poor and uninsured patients with other conditions.

Even if Georgia had agreed to the Medicaid expansion, Grady would still have been hard-pressed to provide the volume and intensity of services these patients need, Haupert said, because direct state funding for mental health services has been reduced across the board.

Nationally, per capita public health spending on mental health services by the state was roughly $120 in 2013. Georgia spent less than half of that, according to data compiled by the Kaiser Family Foundation. It's little wonder then that state and local governments reimburse Grady for only about half of the cost of the services it provides for the uninsured mentally ill.

More than twenty-five patients a day come to Grady's ER with psychiatric symptoms as their primary diagnosis. The hospital's inpatient behavioral health unit has almost tripled in size since 2012. It routinely has 80 percent occupancy and is often too full to take patients from the ER.

Public hospitals around the country report problems similar to Grady's, with other emergencies being crowded out of ERs because of the volume of mentally ill and substance abuse cases, Siegel said.

The American College of Emergency Physicians in 2014 reported that 84 percent of their members said they routinely have to "board" psychiatric patients in the ER—meaning the patients spend at least a day in the ER before a bed on a psychiatric ward became available. Many of those waiting patients— more than 90 percent of them, the ER physicians said—were considered so ill that caring for them in that setting distracted the staff and resulted in reduced services to other ER patients.

Moreover, there is a shortage of beds set aside specifically for emergency psychiatric care in many urban areas. Patients who get admitted may not be able to stay as long as they need to get stabilized and provided with an outpatient treatment plan.

This crisis in deciding who is responsible for treatment and social services for the chronically mentally ill is but the latest iteration in what can best be described as the country's most serious failure in ensuring health care for the poor.

Legacy of Shame

Not surprisingly, at the heart of the dispute is Medicaid, the 1965 program that was supposed to be the safety net for the nation's poor in need of health care.

Prior to Medicaid, states were primarily responsible for mental health care for the poor. They did this with institutions that served mostly to warehouse the severely ill and keep them off the streets. And while there have been periodic reports of neglect and abuse in these institutions—reports that famously started with reformer Dorothea Dix's scathing reports on the conditions of private insane asylums in Massachusetts, New Jersey, Pennsylvania, and other states in the 1840s—many state mental hospitals around the country continue to be plagued by staffing and housing issues that jeopardize patient safety.

With the creation of Medicaid, that division of duties between the states and federal government was fundamentally altered in a way that still has major repercussions for the poor. And it bears closer examination when considering what is happening today.

This newest wave of deinstitutionalized care also differs from the first round of state-owned mental hospital closings in the 1960s and '70s. New antipsychotic drugs and treatment methods developed during that time were thought to make institutional care nearly obsolete.

Even mental health advocates and civil libertarians argued in the courts and at state legislatures that poor, chronically mentally ill patients should be able to receive their care in the least restrictive environment possible, once they had been stabilized in a hospital.

That movement led to closing state mental hospitals around the country over the 1970s and 1980s. Local communities, faced with paying for some of the services that had once been paid for by the state, created community mental health programs. But the money spent on these programs, and the intensity of services they provided to the chronically ill, never matched the need. Nor did it match what the state had been spending on keeping those state hospitals operating before shutting them down.

Moreover, many of the community-based programs were contracted out to providers who seemed more interested in serving the "worried well"—those in need of psychological counseling and assistance with less severe forms of behavioral issues. It's no secret that the services for these types of patients are less intensive and more likely to be covered by conventional health insurance.

Still, that first round of closings established a trend line in public spending on mental health that has shown up with a vengeance now.

Shutting down state hospitals and moving just a portion of the money that had been spent on them to local communities provided states a quick and relatively painless way to save money during times of fiscal austerity. Around the country, state health care spending for mental health declined by 30 percent from 1955 to 1995, a period during which spending on other health services skyrocketed.

The result was that the chronically ill—especially those who were poor and uninsured and who had little or no family resources to draw on—wound up cycling through the wards of the dwindling number of state institutions that stayed open.

Nationwide, the number of beds at state-owned facilities declined by more than 7,000 from 2005 to 2010. Because of budget cuts, no state in 2010 was able now to meet the minimum number of beds deemed adequate for psychiatric services, Siegel said. (The minimum, according to the Treatment Advocacy Center, is 50 beds per 100,000 population.)

From 2009 to 2011 alone, Siegel said, state budget makers around the country cut $1.6 billion in funding for mental health services, despite the fact that demand for those services continues to increase.

And with less state money going to institutionalized care, the inevitable happened. Chronic staffing shortages, poor training, and inadequate monitoring of severely ill patients still stuck inside institutions led to death and abuse.

In Georgia alone, more than a hundred patients died in state hospitals between 2002 and 2006 in what were described as "suspicious circumstances," connected to staffing problems. Additionally, there were nearly two hundred cases of sexual and physical abuse of patients in state hospitals during that time, according to an investigation by the *Atlanta Journal-Constitution*. Incredibly, this was taking place when the state was repeatedly warned about overcrowding and inadequate treatment and supervision, the newspaper reported.

Thankfully, not many states were as bad as Georgia. But in dozens of states, advocates went to the federal courts with similar claims of poor treatment and abuse.

Rather than litigate their obvious failures and have to pay millions in damages, the states secured consent decrees from federal judges with promises that they would do better. Not surprisingly, the result was a new round of closings at some of the worst state-owned facilities and a renewed push for funding that would have been spent on the closed hospitals to go instead to local providers, like Grady.

The Need for Coordinated, Consistent Care

The idea that mental health services can be delivered more effectively in the community rather than in a state institution sounds good, and there is science to back it up. But it requires coordination and consistent funding, which is lacking in many states and localities.

A large study of Illinois patients shows that those being treated by ACT teams (like the team at Grady) cost about $10,000 per patient per year—not much more than the cost of a single ER visit and a seven-day stay in the psychiatric unit.

The study showed that many of these patients would wind up in the ER and hospitalized two or three times a year. Providing better services in the community and keeping them out of the hospital saves money in the long run. Moreover, those who are disabled and qualify for Medicaid often wind up in nursing homes, where the cost of care is higher than it would be if the patient is stable and living independently, Illinois advocates found.

This last finding—about the provision of mental health services in nursing homes—bears further examination, because it illustrates how many states have developed ways to maximize federal dollars for Medicaid services while at the same time minimizing state spending on public programs that have traditionally fallen under the auspices of state and local governments.

Some policy analysts have adopted a term, *transinstitutionalization*, to describe how states have moved mentally ill patients from state-owned institutions to privately owned nursing homes where their care is paid for with Medicaid. Richard Frank, an economics professor at the Harvard Medical School, was among the first to fully articulate what happened.

Not surprisingly, it involves Medicaid.

In 1965, when Medicaid was created, it was designed as a multifaceted insurance plan providing coverage to low-income families and elderly Americans who could no longer work and for whom Social Security income and Medicare was inadequate for basic medical needs, including long-term care in nursing homes.

Curiously, federal policy makers specifically exempted state-run mental institutions from qualifying for Medicaid reimbursement for the services they were providing for the poor. This happened despite the fact that state mental institutions were, by far, the largest component of public mental health spending in the 1960s.

The thinking then may have been that these large publicly owned facilities provided little in the way of real medical services. Instead, they were viewed as "custodial" institutions where the mentally ill were taken when there was no place else for them to go.

Clearly, there were budgetary reasons for exempting state mental hospitals too. If patients in state mental hospitals were covered by Medicaid, the cost of the program to the federal budget would have skyrocketed, perhaps two to three times higher than initial projections for the entire program, according to one accounting.

So Congress and federal officials wrote regulations limiting Medicaid reimbursements to traditional, acute-care hospitals, which offered inpatient services that lasted just long enough to stabilize patients and discharge them with medications to help control their illness. The theory was that Medicaid enrollees would have a choice of where to get their care: private hospital mental health units and in nursing homes, if they could not care for themselves after they were discharged.

By 1972, a change in Medicaid eligibility opened the door for states to shift some of their costs for mental health care on to the federal government. That was the year Congress approved Medicaid funding for people who were on Supplemental Security Income, or SSI because of physical or mental disabilities.

Thus, Medicaid became the primary payer of health care services for two distinctly different populations. The first group was people enrolled in Temporary Assistance to Needy Families (TANF), a population that largely consists of single women and their young children. The second group includes those enrolled in Supplemental Security Income (SSI), a population that includes the long-term disabled and elderly poor.

People on TANF have somewhat higher rates of treatment for mental conditions than the population in general, but budget makers did not think it would have a huge impact on Medicaid funding. They were largely correct.

The other group of newly eligible Medicaid enrollees, the SSI population, was a much different story, as it turned out.

Medicaid spending on mental health services for SSI recipients proved to be two to three times higher than for individuals and families on welfare. Moreover, this disabled population needs a variety of other health services, all of which are also covered by Medicaid.

The result is that fully one quarter of all SSI enrollees between the ages of eighteen and sixty-four are getting mental health services paid for by Medicaid, accounting for more than a third of all Medicaid spending. This group has represented the fastest-growing group of SSI enrollees since the late 1980s, making Medicaid an important payer for perhaps the most impaired people with mental health conditions in the country.

Moreover, making SSI recipients eligible for Medicaid altered the way states traditionally provided, and paid for, such services for the poor and uninsured.

A number of studies have linked the per capita rise of nursing home beds in states to a corresponding decline in state spending on mental hospitals. The implication behind this kind of transinstitutionalization is that states were more than happy to see poor elderly patients—who made up the largest portion of the population in state mental hospitals in the 1960s and 1970s—being cared for (and paid for largely with federal Medicaid dollars) in nursing homes instead.

Nor have many states been shy about shifting some of the cost of direct mental health services from their own budgets to Medicaid.

This has been especially problematic in the checkered history of locally operated mental health "systems" that were supposed to pick up the care of the poor in the community when they were discharged from state hospitals.

These community health systems, often operated by private nonprofit contractors, have the responsibility to serve both the Medicaid population and the poor who do not qualify for Medicaid. The cost of care for this last group is considered the responsibility of state and local governments, which usually provide grants to pay the contractors to provide the services.

Some states applied the cost of these grants toward their "match" for overall Medicaid spending, meaning that even though total state spending on mental health may rise, the federal government was picking up a larger portion of it and minimizing the impact on state taxpayers.

State mental health officials around the country had a description for this practice: "If it moves, Medicaid it." By doing so, they were not abusing the law; they were merely taking advantage of an available financing mechanism.

Nor was moving patients who had been in the state-run system to contract providers where Medicaid would pay for their care a flawed policy. Remember, prior to Medicaid, the state had been responsible for covering care for these patients in state institutions entirely out of the state budget. Now the cost was being split between the state and federal government, with the Feds covering at least half of the cost and often much more.

What's important is what the states did with their savings thanks to the switch.

Many used the money to either expand Medicaid eligibility or to provide more state-funded mental health services directly to people who could not qualify for Medicaid and could not afford to pay for the care themselves.

But Georgia did neither.

Like several other states in the South, Georgia decided to use the money it had been spending on mental health services elsewhere in the state budget.

Predictably, the patient census in many state institutions began to decline. But the demand for mental health services— from low-income people not covered by Medicaid or SSI—did not go away.

The New Mental Institutions: Streets, Jails and Public Hospitals

Most of the poor and uninsured were simply left out of the system altogether, despite the fact that many of them had severe forms of illness and significant impairment. Many eventually made their way back into some form of government-paid care: state hospitals, prisons, county jails, or public hospitals.

Still, other states decided to take advantage of the 1981 dispro-portionate share hospital law (DSH) designed to pay hospitals that took in a large number of poor and uninsured patients a higher rate of reimbursement for Medicaid and Medicare services.

By 1990, several states successfully argued to federal regula-tors that their state mental institutions should qualify for DSH funding because, by definition, these hospitals were filled with poor and low-income mentally ill patients who were receiving more than custodial care. Still others were able to work around the provisions of the original law that barred Medicaid funding for state-owned mental institutions. There were other examples of cost shifting from state budgets to the federal budget for mental health services.

Again, had these schemes been followed up by using the savings achieved by the states for better-targeted services for the poor and mentally ill, the impact may not have been so severe. But these and other state policies—including low Medicaid reimbursement rates for private psychiatrists that all but encouraged them to shun Medicaid patients—all combined to significantly weaken public mental health services in many states over the past three decades.

Richard Frank of Harvard and other researchers who have studied actions by the states since the enactment of Medicaid have come to conclude that cost shifting fundamentally dis-torted the historic role the states played as being the providers of last resort for low-income and uninsured mentally ill residents.

Instead of improving or expanding services to these vulner-able patients after Medicaid was enacted, the researchers said, many states spent most of their energy trying to find ways for the federal government to pick up more of the costs.

This failure to provide a baseline of appropriate men-tal health care for the poor and uninsured helps explain why scandals inside state mental institutions in Georgia and else-where resulted in lawsuits and court settlements in recent years. Those consent decrees have resulted in a new round of hospital closures and more experiments in contracting for services.

But evidence is mounting that this round of deinstitution-alization will require a much higher level of intensity and better coordination of treatment approaches within the community. State officials should understand, advocates say, that measuring those costs against hospitalization alone doesn't present the full picture, so a meaningful cost comparison is not always possi-ble. Still, coordinated care within a community can work.

Case in point: one in five inmates in local jails and state prisons has a serious mental illness, according to the Bureau of Justice statistics of the US Department of Justice. Most are not a threat to anyone other than themselves. But they are taking up space in jails that ought to be used for those accused of violent crimes.

Moreover, when they finally get before a judge, they often get credit for time served and are released to unstable living arrangements where their condition worsens, and they recycle through the courts or emergency rooms or both.

A handful of localities are taking a more innovative, coor-dinated approach.

In San Antonio, Texas, the courts, jails, police departments, hospitals, and county government leaders decided to pool the money each was spending on services to the mentally ill and coordinate a unified approach to treatment.

Besides creating a dedicated hospital unit and outpa-tient primary care and psychiatric clinic, the Bexar County Restoration Center has programs for detoxification, housing, and job training. The integrated approach, which serves about 18,000 people a year, has saved the county about $10 million annually that it otherwise would have spent on independently run services at the jail, hospital, and other government pro-grams, according to the county.

State legislators and budget makers should not deceive themselves—as many have done in the past—by believing that the state will save money by closing hospital wards and transferring some of the funding to local providers. The demand is great and continues to grow. The goal should not be simply to save money, advocates say. The goal should be more effective care.

By expanding Medicaid to cover people above the poverty level, the way the ACA envisioned, much of the financial burden on states and localities could be relieved.

Given the high prevalence of mental health and substance abuse treatment among the prison and jail population, getting these incarcerated individuals signed up for Medicaid, or enrolling them in the individual insurance marketplace before they finish serving their terms, could mean a significant reduction in the frequent-flyer population cycling through the court system and public hospital emergency rooms.

A Washington State study in 2013 found that the vast majority of the 160,000 inmates released from jails would be eligible for Medicaid expansion if the state took advantage of the federal government's push to enroll individuals with incomes up to 138 percent of the poverty level. More than 120,000 inmates had no state-funded health care coverage at all, the study found.

Long-standing federal regulations do not allow inmates serving time for crimes to be covered by Medicaid while they are incarcerated. It leaves the decision up to the states about whether to terminate these individuals from Medicaid, or suspend them while they are jailed. (This is another reason why public hospitals often shoulder the burden for acute care of jailed prisoners. In their contracts with local governments, many public hospitals agree to provide this care for free or at a substantial discount in return for tax support for their operations.)

The ACA, however, encourages states to apply for Medicaid for inmates while they are incarcerated so that they might have coverage once they are released and reduce the risk of recidivism due to behavioral health issues.

These patients need a range of services at the local level that extends well beyond monitoring their medications and making sure they make their appointments. Almost all of them require intensive case management, like the kind offered at Grady, for a minimum of two to three years.

Yet the resources to support this intervention will predictably never be found in the many states, like Georgia, that have refused Medicaid expansion.

The cost of providing health care services to mentally ill and addicted inmates will be borne instead by state and local taxpayers. All the worse, Georgia's official policy is that no state institution or state employee is allowed to assist residents— jailed or free—in signing up for the insurance marketplaces under the ACA. That effectively prohibits jail workers from helping prisoners find and pay for the care they need once they are released.

Unfortunately, such shortsightedness has become the norm for how too many states care for the most vulnerable population in need of mental health services—those who are in jail as well as those who are trying to survive on the streets.

About half of the estimated five thousand homeless people in Atlanta are thought to be mentally ill or addicted to drugs, alcohol, or both. Many of them would qualify for Medicaid if Georgia agreed to expansion. They rely instead on the street-level care they get from Mercy Care, the city's largest provider of primary care services for the homeless.

Mercy Care gets no state or local funding to speak of. More than 90 percent of the patients it sees do not have insurance. It relies on charitable contributions and federal grants to carry out its mission.

At times, the demand is overwhelming, Mercy Care's staff said.

That means Grady's thirteenth-floor psych unit will stay crowded; the names on the community treatment team's whiteboard will only grow; and county jails along with state prisons will continue to house mentally ill Americans lost in one of the nation's worst public health failures.

10

TRAUMA CARE: THE SERVICE
WE TAKE FOR GRANTED

Dr. Omar Danner spends much of his day waiting for elevators and running the stairways of Grady Memorial Hospital.

His office is clustered with those of the other attending surgeons on the seventh floor, not too far away from the surgical intensive care unit. The operating rooms are on the next floor down. Grady's Level 1 trauma unit is on the ground floor, eight floors away when he is in his office, but seventeen floors down if he is on the top floor of the building, where there is a fitness center for use by the medical staff.

"I try to get up there whenever I can," said Dr. Danner, a tall, barrel-chested man. "Sometimes I need to let off a little steam."

Dr. Danner looks as if he could snap you in half in an angry moment, but he seldom raises his voice. His colleagues say he never loses his composure, even when all hell is breaking loose around him.

Perfect for a trauma surgeon, they say.

On average, he works sixty to a hundred hours a week, more than half of which is spent taking care of critically injured trauma patients. A native of Birmingham, one of the first African-Americans to enroll at the University of Alabama Medical School, Dr. Danner has played an outsized role in some of Grady's most difficult trauma cases.

It wasn't on his original career path to end up at Grady, or even as a trauma surgeon. After surgical, critical care and trauma training at The Johns Hopkins Hospital in Baltimore, he completed a fellowship at University of Pittsburgh Medical Center in one of the country's top training programs in advanced minimally invasive surgery—the kind where the doctor uses a lighted scope to illuminate the surgical site within the body and remove diseased tissue, or remove internal organs by sucking them through button-sized holes in the skin. General surgery was where he thought he wanted to be.

He was in private surgical practice in Charlotte doing just that for a short stint before he realized something was missing: excitement, fulfillment and "intellectual stimulation," he said.

He found what he was looking for when he joined the Morehouse School of Medicine faculty and set up his practice at Grady. He's a fixture there now, teaching a new corps of young physicians every year, supervising trauma fellowships, and keeping detailed records about trauma unit patients and their outcomes. In his spare time, he's active in a mentoring program called Reach One, Each One for minority high school students interested in medical science.

"There's an adrenaline rush with trauma," Dr. Danner said. "You are there for a very clear reason, to save a life, even though you may never have met the patient on your table. Your first job is to get and keep the patient stable. It takes a team to do that. And only then can you think about what you have to do surgically. That's what makes it exciting."

If there is a defining medical service of America's large public hospitals—a singular characteristic that identifies them in their communities—it is trauma. The association began early, when surgeons at the nation's oldest public hospital, Bellevue in New York City, met horse-drawn wagons arriving with severely injured patients at the front door.

Today, medical helicopters transport thousands of patients with life-threatening injuries every year to designated trauma centers. They come by air from the carnage on roads hundreds of miles away or, more often, via ground ambulances squeezing through the emergency lanes of gridlocked metro Interstates.

American hospitals admit more than two million patients

per year due to trauma. Nearly 200,000 Americans lose their lives each year because of traumatic injury, making it the leading cause of death for people under the age of forty-five.

Grady handles about 3,500 trauma cases a year—more patients than are admitted for all causes to dozens of other Georgia hospitals in any year. Often, these "trucks"—as emergency responders call them—are hauling the victims and sometimes the perpetrators of gunshots, stabbings, and other violent acts.

The modern medicine practiced in America's trauma centers is the result of decades of surgical science and born out of battlefield innovations at field hospitals dating from the Civil War to the conflicts in Iraq and Afghanistan. Under the best of practices, trauma services are part of a coordinated network of hospitals within a region, each with varying levels of care and expertise well beyond what can be provided in emergency rooms.

The R Adams Cowley Shock Trauma Center, part of the University of Maryland Medical Center and the leader of a statewide trauma network, is a one-hundred-bed trauma hospital. It is also the place where many of the nation's best trauma surgeons and physicians have trained.

A large and coordinated team of medical professionals is required to stop bleeding, stabilize vital signs, and protect the heart, the brain, and other organs from long-term damage even before trauma surgery commences. Few hospitals can stage the choreography needed to pull it off. Nor are most areas of the country served by a trauma network as coordinated as Maryland's.

To do it requires extraordinary training of nurses, round-the-clock availability of specialty doctors, separate facilities from the more routine cases handled in the emergency room, and the ability to gain access, quickly, to sophisticated and expensive imaging equipment like CT, MRI, and PET scanners. There is a certification process that rates the hospital's ability to provide the service. Getting a designation as Level 1, the most intensive, is the hardest to achieve. Most hospitals in the United States that have trauma center designations are Level 3 or below.

From a cost perspective, the trauma unit is usually the most expensive place in the hospital. Patients cared for in these units run up bills in the tens of thousands of dollars per day and often spend months in the intensive care unit recovering from their injuries.

Unfortunately, many of them—especially the crime and mayhem cases—don't bring insurance cards with them. That's why public hospitals, most of which are chartered by local or state government to accept all comers, have traditionally taken on the Level 1 trauma challenge. They have the resident staff of medical specialists on hand around the clock. Plus, since many of them are teaching hospitals, they have a research and education mission that helps disseminate information about what works and what doesn't. For decades, public hospitals were the sole trauma providers.

But with competition for patients increasing in the 1980s and early 1990s, a number of community hospitals entered the trauma world.

In Atlanta, marketing experts encouraged hospital administrators to offer the service as a way of advancing their hospitals' reputation. "They were looking for a halo effect," said Dr. Thomas M. Scalea, physician in chief at Maryland Shock Trauma. "For a while everyone seemed to want to get into the business. But they didn't know how expensive it was to keep going." Some set up helicopter services on their rooftops to scoop up accident victims on the Interstate and bring them back for treatment.

They made arrangements for neurosurgeons and other specialists to be on call, even if they weren't in the hospital. They produced slick television commercials to boast of their expertise and service to the community. Most of the new entrants to the field were designated by the American College of Surgeons as Level 2 or Level 3 centers, but the larger Level 1 centers seemed happy to have them share some of the load.

Unfortunately, the commitment didn't last long. Many insurance policies didn't cover the full cost of the service, or the patients they did cover maxed out their lifetime benefits very quickly. It was nearly impossible to find the revenue needed to keep many trauma units going, much less absorb the cost of long-term hospitalization for the uninsured patients who survived, Dr. Scalea said.

In Georgia, trauma centers asked the state for money to help them survive. (Maryland, the leader in trauma service, does this, but most states don't.) Instead, the state established a coordinating network to help manage some of the data collection and record keeping hospitals needed to maintain their trauma status.

It wasn't enough. Within a decade, most of them gave it up. There was much more money to be made expanding cancer treatments and cardiovascular services, especially with the explosion of angioplasty procedures taking place at the time.

The lack of an adequate trauma network got so bad that in 2010, the Georgia general assembly asked voters in a ballot initiative to put a $10 per year fee on their auto-license renewals to help offset some of the costs for hospitals offering trauma service. The fee would have generated about $80 million yearly for the trauma providers to share. But the voters said no, leaving Grady in Atlanta and public hospitals in Macon, Augusta, and Savannah as the only Level 1 trauma centers in the largest state (in land mass) west of the Mississippi River.

Indeed, the lack of Level 1 trauma care in wide swaths of the country has generated concern in public health circles. The failure to get critically injured patients to adequate trauma care within the first hour of their injuries results in about seven hundred deaths per year in Georgia alone, according to the American College of Surgeons.

A similar scenario played out in Florida, where twenty-one of the state's designated trauma centers shut down in the 1980s and 1990s.

But in the fast-changing health care marketplace, interest in trauma care is heating up again. The reasons for this reemergence of trauma vary from state to state. Florida, for instance, has some state funding available for trauma care, thanks to vehicle-registration taxes and fines from red-light cameras being earmarked for the service. Other states have started subsidizing trauma care in other ways. But one thing is becoming clear: by accepting the right patients with the right injuries, trauma care could possibly turn a profit.

As the population ages, the life-threatening condition that comes through the nation's emergency medical services networks the most is injury from falls, with many of the victims being treated by trauma centers, according to Dr. Scalea. While the popular image of trauma centers involves saving the lives of victims of gunshot wounds or car crashes, most of the patients being treated at lower-level trauma centers are there because they fell at home or on the job and needed the expertise of trauma doctors to care for their head or spinal injuries. Not coincidentally, they are also the patients most likely to be covered by health insurance.

Plus, hospitals have found new ways to bill for the service—in some cases, levying a "trauma activation fee" of $25,000 to $30,000 the moment a trauma patient comes through the doors. They can collect the fee even if the patient is only stabilized and moved on to a higher-level trauma hospital.

This renewed trauma interest seems fueled, at least in part, by for-profit hospitals in large metro markets, especially in Florida, Texas, and California, where HCA, the nation's largest hospital chain, is leading the charge. Of the nearly two hundred trauma centers that opened nationwide between 2009 and 2012, only a handful of them are in underserved rural areas. Most are in suburban communities.

And, as is often the case with changes in health policy and the private insurance marketplace, Dr. Scalea and others have concerns that urban public hospitals—and their nonpaying Level 1 trauma patients—will be left behind as yet another profit-seeking wave washes through the nation's $3 trillion health care marketplace.

That's because the nation's best trauma hospitals, like Grady, have to be open all the time to all patients—from supermodels injured in car wrecks to street thugs stabbed in gang warfare. To do it, they must offset their losses by treating an adequate volume of insured patients. Patients like Richard Beckel, whom we met in the Introduction and learn more about next, and Sylvia Ennis whose story appears in this chapter. These are patients who never thought they would wind up at Grady Memorial Hospital.

Two Patients, One Doctor: Their Stories
Richard Beckel

When you fly into Atlanta, it's hard to tell from the air how big the city really is. A tree canopy, even in the winter, masks the city's many wonderful neighborhoods. Even in car-crazed Atlanta, where single-occupancy vehicles rule the day, these neighborhoods are ideal for walking, as the sidewalks are filled on good-weather days with people pushing baby strollers and dogs pulling on their masters' leashes.

West Wesley Road snakes through Buckhead, one of Atlanta's most exclusive neighborhoods. It crosses over Interstate 75 and Peachtree Road before coming to a halt in the heart of Buckhead's commercial district. Cyclists love it because the route is not always crowded like other parts of Buckhead, and the scenery includes stately homes with colorful landscaping.

Still, bicycling West Wesley can be dangerous. It has

narrow, two-lane sections, and in Atlanta, drivers of autos and trucks often assume primacy on the roadway. When you are on a bike, there is little room for error.

On a Sunday afternoon in February 2012, Richard Beckel planned to ride twenty to thirty miles before he and his wife, Isobel Moutrey, went to a Super Bowl party later that evening. He and a neighbor took off on their bicycles as they often did on weekends when the weather was nice. They headed for Buckhead, a few miles away from their homes in the up-and-coming west side of Atlanta, where new housing developments are claiming vacant lots and underdeveloped tracts near the city's sprawling railroad yards.

It was about 4:00 p.m. when they got to West Wesley.

Richard Beckel never saw the driver who hit him. His GT Road Bike went one way and Richard the other. He slammed into the front of the car, tumbled across the windshield, was catapulted forty feet through the air, and landed on his back on the asphalt pavement.

It was a wonder he wasn't killed instantly. The helmet he always wore probably saved his life. Miraculously, he did not immediately lose consciousness.

His neighbor riding with him got to him quickly and tried to keep him conscious. Other drivers stopped to offer assistance. So did homeowners on West Wesley, bringing blankets to keep him warm.

Someone in the crowd that had gathered called 911. His neighbor borrowed a phone from a bystander and told his wife to ask another neighborhood couple to get Richard's wife, Isobel, and take her to Grady. A Grady EMS crew had already arrived and stabilized Richard for blunt trauma. As they put him in the ambulance, everyone was concerned for his survival.

On her way to the hospital, Isobel thought: "Why Grady?" Richard had suffered a severe concussion two years early while working in their yard. He had been taken to Piedmont Hospital nearest to where they lived. They were great at Piedmont. Piedmont was also closest to the site of the accident. "Why Grady?"

When she got there, the first thing she noticed about the big public hospital's emergency department was that security stopped her and made her go through metal detectors. It infuriated her. What kind of place is this?

"What the hell?" she said. "My husband is back there, and you are going to make me strip down for a metal detector? I started throwing my purse, my shoulder bag—everything I had with me—on the conveyor belt. I just wanted to get back there and find out what was happening to Richard."

For forty-five minutes, maybe an hour, Isobel sat in the crowded, noisy ER waiting room, still unsure of the extent of her husband's injuries.

One of her neighbors suggested she tell the triage nurse that Richard had suffered head concussion a few years ago. Perhaps that would speed things along, she recalled. To her surprise, it worked. They ushered her to a hallway outside the ER where she waited, this time by herself.

Two doctors came to speak with her. One of them was Dr. Omar Danner, the trauma surgeon. The news was not good. Richard's injuries were life threatening. He needed surgery as soon as possible, but he was not stable enough yet to survive it.

Someone handed her Richard's wedding band. It was a "brutal" moment of realization, Isobel said, when she first realized her husband might indeed die.

Two nurses from the unit brought her to Richard's bedside. She held his hand and saw him move his leg—a good sign that he wasn't paralyzed, she thought, and she assured him he would be okay.

They escorted her to a waiting room across the hallway, just outside the ER. By this time, Richard's mother, Peggy Beckel, and several friends and family members had joined her. Before he was taken to surgery, Isobel took his mother to his side.

It was then she caught a glimpse of what was going on in trauma. She described it later as organized chaos. Doctors and nurses were surrounding Richard's gurney. Lights, monitors, blinking instrument panels. Alarms were going off everywhere. Blood was ordered; IV bags were on poles and held aloft in nurses' hands. Each team member seemed to have a specific job to do.

Isobel was pulled aside by several surgeons while Richard's mother was with him. One was asking for some more medical history for her husband; the others were telling her that they were confident Richard had no lasting paralysis. Richard was still conscious. His mother told her that Richard apologized to her for causing her to worry.

Everything that happened in the trauma unit, every utterance by a doctor, every rushed procedure and every new code called out for another specialist to come to his side, Isobel tried to measure as either good news or bad. In fact it was a little of both.

The trauma specialist had seen injuries like this before—motorcycle riders thrown to the pavement from their bikes, hikers who stumbled and fell down the side of a mountain, passengers in cars who were thrown out of the vehicle in major crashes. They were all bruised and battered on the outside, with clear evidence of broken bones and bleeding like crazy on the inside.

There's a reason why they call it blunt trauma.

Dr. Danner could tell his patient would need massive abdominal surgery. The tachycardia he was experiencing—the abnormally fast and hard-to-control heart rhythm—was a sign of an additional injury of some sort to the heart. The contusions on Richard's body showed his sternum was cracked.

About 8:30 p.m., he was wheeled into surgery. It would be seven hours, and three different surgeries later, before Richard left the OR. During this time Dr. Danner brought Isobel some good news. Richard had survived, but they were still concerned about his irregular, rapid heartbeat that had yet to be brought under control. They were considering some other procedures.

Dr. Danner said he had to resect the colon as well as deal

with damage to Richard's spleen, kidneys, and other organs. Ribs on both sides of Richard's body were broken or crushed. His collarbone was broken. The left distal radius was smashed, as was his left femur (broken arm, broken leg). There was damage to his upper spine and bone fragments in the spinal canal. There were serious contusions to his lungs, and one of the arteries of his heart was torn. He was still on a ventilator to help him breathe.

Isobel was taken to an intensive care unit waiting room. The overhead television in the waiting room was constantly on, and no one could seem to find the remote control to lower the volume. From time to time, one of the hospital volunteers would turn it down by poking it with a yardstick. She remembers smelling marijuana on the clothes of some of the people in the waiting room. There was vomit on the restroom floor.

In the weeks Richard was hospitalized, Isobel spent time in several Grady waiting rooms, meeting family members of patients being treated there for gunshot wounds and stabbings. A few had been flown to Grady from other parts of the state, so these waiting rooms became their second home.

Isobel got to know many of them and rejoiced with them when their loved ones were allowed to leave the ICU. Richard's dependency on the ventilator and other complications kept him from leaving the ICU.

While in the ICU, Richard needed a tracheotomy—an operation to place the ventilator through an incision in the throat directly into his upper airway. He stayed on the ventilator for weeks. He developed a urinary tract infection that was difficult to treat. He contracted pneumonia, a routine complication in such cases. His kidneys started to fail. His heart would go back into tachycardia inexplicably from time to time, requiring drugs to stabilize it and reduce the risk of stroke and heart attack.

An important moment came weeks into his hospitalization when Dr. Kenneth Wilson, then the Morehouse School of Medicine's chief of trauma at Grady, was able to wean Richard from the ventilator.

Just over six weeks after his Sunday bike ride nearly killed him, Richard Beckel left the Grady ICU and was taken to the Shepherd Center in Atlanta, which specializes in orthopedic and spinal injuries. The bill for his hospital care at Grady alone toppled $1 million. Luckily for him, and for Grady, he had insurance.

Sylvia Ennis

Sylvia Ennis was pumped for her first day at work after the Christmas and New Year's holidays as she got in her car to go to her job at Emory University, east of Atlanta. "I felt good. I was looking good too. I had on a new skirt, some new shoes and earrings. It was going to be a good day."

But just as her two-minute commute commenced—as she buckled up her seat belt—a six-inch-diameter branch of the huge pine tree that towered over her car broke away and crashed through the windshield of her Toyota. The heavy branch bent the steering wheel, pierced Sylvia through the abdomen, and exited below her tailbone. As she sat there in the front seat, stunned by what had just happened, she thought, "I'm going to die today."

People rushed to her side not knowing what to do, or even whether to try and move her. Electric lines brought down by the tree limb were perilously close to her and the car. A 911 call was made. People asked Sylvia if there was anyone she wanted them to call. At first, she couldn't think of an answer. Then she remembered her sister's phone number. As the minutes ticked by, she realized something else: "I'm breathing. I'm still alive."

The emergency medical responders got her out of the car even though she was still impaled by the pine branch. They transported her that way because they feared removing it at the scene would result in massive bleeding from wounds they could not see. She was conscious and alert.

It was a smart move.

The morning Ennis arrived at the Grady trauma center, Dr. Omar Danner was on trauma call, conducting rounds on surgical recovery patients when he was paged to get to the trauma unit immediately. He had a hard time getting an elevator ride downstairs from his office. There are supposed to be special elevators for doctors to use for exactly this purpose, but they are often busy, sometimes not available at all. And the general elevators used by the public at Grady are always crowded and tend to stop at almost every floor. All Dr. Danner knew was that a bad trauma case was arriving, and he needed to get there quickly. This time he ran down the stairs.

"I'd never seen anything like it," he said, when he examined Ennis in the trauma center and saw the tree limb had "harpooned" her.

The immediate problem that Wednesday morning was that Sylvia's blood pressure had tanked. It was too low to get an intravenous line placed or even draw blood work. Dr. Danner ordered a transfusion and took her to the OR, where a team of anesthesiology specialists intubated her so that she could breathe. Next, intravenous lines were placed. The team slowly reestablished her blood pressure and waited for her to stabilize. Only then could they start the surgery, and "at that point we would have to make up the operation as we went along," Dr. Danner said. (Weeks later, after Sylvia had recovered and he could joke about it, Dr. Danner told his colleagues that he was pressed into service that day as a general surgeon, a trauma surgeon, and a tree surgeon.)

The tree limb had ripped through her abdominal wall, shredding the muscles and slicing her intestines and other internal organs. They were a mess. "We have to triage where the worst bleeding was first, stop it, and move on to the next spot," Dr. Danner remembers telling himself. "We just need to get her through this and stabilize her," he told the trauma surgery team. More detailed surgical repairs to her injured organs could be done later.

The initial operation took three hours, but Dr. Danner and his team got the bleeding stopped. Over the next six weeks, Sylvia would be monitored carefully for internal bleeding, her intestines reconstucted and then a new series of surgeries would be staged at appropriate intervals to repair the damaged abdominal wall and other injuries. She was in the hospital for three months. All her organs were saved.

Sylvia Ennis remembers waking up after surgery to "all these faces of handsome doctors and nurses surrounding me." Later, she recalled, "They were the faces of the people who saved my life."

Much later, she remembered what she thought when the EMTs put her in the ambulance that morning and told her, even though they were only a few blocks from Emory University Hospital, they were taking her to Grady.

"Oh, Grady," she recalled thinking to herself. It was as much an acknowledgment that her condition was serious as it was some concern that, if she was lucky enough to live, she would no doubt be spending a lot of time there.

Blunt versus Penetrating Trauma: Why It Matters

You hear that mixed review of Grady around Atlanta a lot. For several years the hospital gave away bumper stickers that read, "If I'm in an accident take me to Grady." To which many Atlantans reading the stickers would quickly add, "And then when I am better, get me the hell out of there."

Supermodel Niki Taylor, whose youthful face graced more than 250 magazine covers by the time she was twenty-five years of age, wound up at Grady in April 2001 when the car she was riding in slammed into a utility pole on Atlanta streets. She lost

80 percent of her blood volume. Her liver was torn in half. It took forty surgeries and eight weeks to repair the damage.

She left Grady for her home in Florida, having never heard of it before she arrived, yet thankful for its expertise. She said she wanted to help the hospital—which was losing millions of dollars a year at the time—raise money to stay solvent.

Richard Beckel and Sylvia Ennis have had similar conversions about Georgia's largest charity hospital. They can be seen on public service advertisements touting how "Atlanta can't live without Grady." They help raise awareness about the critical need for trauma and other services that only Grady can provide.

But their cases, as dramatic as they were, do not make the newscasts as often as those of other trauma patients who rely on Grady—not just the victims but sometimes the perpetrators injured in violent crime. Footage of ambulances backing up to the trauma doors at Grady often dominates the opening segment of morning newscasts after a particularly bad night of crime. "The victim was taken to Grady" may be the most widely used string of six words on Atlanta television.

It could also be an explanation for why—despite the proven need for taxpayer help—Grady routinely gets shortchanged by state government in Georgia. Unlike several other states, Georgia does not provide direct taxpayer funding to trauma hospitals for patient care, perhaps because the public seems to believe that too many of its trauma patients are undeserving of the service.

Not only did voters turn down the modest effort to assess a fee on auto licenses to pay for trauma care, the state's politicians have steadfastly refused to expand Medicaid eligibility for Georgians working in low-paying jobs where they aren't covered by insurance.

So when poor and uninsured Georgians need trauma care, the hospitals that provide it are on the hook for unpaid bills. In 2010 the annual tab for uncompensated trauma care in Georgia topped $250 million.

Administrators at Grady and the other major trauma centers in the state had hoped that with the 2010 passage of the Affordable Care Act—as more Georgians gained private insurance through the new, subsidized exchanges—some of the uncompensated care load would be lifted. And indeed it has.

But without the Medicaid expansion, the future of trauma care remains anything but certain. Public hospitals in Florida are up against it as well. Despite the governor's onetime interest in expanding Medicaid, the legislature refuses to do so. And Texas—with the largest percentage of uninsured residents in the country—has also refused to expand Medicaid, leaving its Level 1 trauma centers at financial risk as lower-level centers siphon off paying customers.

Moreover, the contentious and ongoing debate in Congress over Obamacare has directly impacted trauma in ways few people even know about.

The 2010 law called for the creation of about fifty "discretionary" programs designed to stimulate state action to improve health services as the law was being implemented. They are considered discretionary because Congress has to agree on a funding level for each of them in the annual appropriation process.

But the larger issues surrounding the law itself—the creation of state exchanges, the individual mandate, and Medicaid expansion—made these relatively small initiatives easy to ignore. Indeed, as the law was being contested before the Supreme Court in 2012 and debated in the presidential election that same year, in the midterm elections in 2014 and before the high court again the following year, most of them never got funded.

Four of the initiatives involved trauma care, including federal grants that could be used by states to help cover some of the financial losses that trauma centers incur from nonpaying patients. Another program could have been used to provide direct federal funding to vital trauma centers that were in imminent threat of shutting down.

Despite the uncertainty of government funding at both the federal and state level, some hospitals appear to be banking on the marketplace and getting back into the trauma business. The vast majority of the new trauma centers that have opened in recent years are Level 2 or below—meaning that they usually don't handle the most extreme cases. Indeed, under loose regulations in a few states, some are not much more than specially equipped emergency rooms, where the most severely injured trauma cases can be stabilized and transferred to Level 1 trauma centers.

Normally, this renewed interest in providing trauma care would be considered an encouraging development. But in the delicate balancing act of how and where trauma care is available, how it is paid for, and who is available to provide it, the new competition for the service is raising concerns, especially among the urban public hospitals that have carried the load for so many years.

Expanding the vital service to areas that lack it is one thing, but that's not what appears to be happening. The new centers are cropping up, not surprisingly, in suburban areas of big cities.

Just across Interstate 75/85 from Grady, the Atlanta Medical Center, a for-profit hospital owned by Tenet Healthcare, asked for and received Level 1 trauma designation in 2011. WellStar Kennestone Hospital, a nonprofit public hospital in the northwest suburb of Marietta, became a Level 2 center the following year. Kennestone had been a trauma center in the 1980s, but dropped out of the network a few years later. Atlanta Medical Center had dropped to Level 2 status, but now moved back up. Why the change of heart?

Two words: Blunt trauma.

Of the two kinds of trauma victims to routinely come into hospitals—those suffering from internal injuries (blunt) and those who are bleeding from gunshot wounds and stabbings (penetrating)—the blunt trauma patients are the best insured. The vast majority of them are there due to falls. Many of them are elderly people who fell at home and are covered by Medicare.

Automobile accident victims in suburban areas suffering from blunt trauma are also more likely to be covered by health insurance, or by liability insurance through their auto-insurance carriers, or that of the person responsible for the wreck. Moreover, under the ACA, there is no maximum yearly or lifetime limit on paying out benefits for coverage. (Prior to 2014, private insurance coverage often had a $250,000 or $500,000 maximum lifetime benefit, which trauma patients can go through fast, leaving the hospital to absorb the remaining bills.)

Significantly, as hospitals and insurers negotiate new contracts for reimbursement for all services under the ACA, some are forming networks that require beneficiaries to go to certain hospitals for heart surgery, cancer care, and now even trauma. Patients who go out of network for these services have to pay more out of their own pockets.

The first sign of potential problems with the new era of insured trauma care took place in late 2014 in a dispute between Blue Cross and Blue Shield of Georgia—by far Georgia's largest insurer—and Grady.

At the heart of the dispute was Blue Cross and Blue Shield's demand that Grady agree to in-network negotiated rates. If Grady balked, the hospital would be declared out of network, and patients covered by Blue Cross and Blue Shield of Georgia would have to pay much more out of their own pockets if they went to Grady for any service, not just trauma. And with the Atlanta Medical Center near Grady offering Level 1 trauma care, Blue Cross patients could stay in-network and not face high out-of-pocket expenses.

It wasn't an idle threat. Blue Cross covers many more Georgians than any other insurer, including, at the time, an exclusive contract for the state's 600,000 government employees, their dependents, and state retirees. Nevertheless, in late

November 2014, Grady failed to negotiate a new contract so Blue Cross declared the state's largest public hospital out of network.

The hospital quickly mounted a major media campaign to let the public know about the dispute, calling on the insurance giant to be fair to Grady. The state legislature, not always Grady's biggest promoter, decided to get involved in the dispute because of the large number of state employees it would impact.

The issue they chose to highlight was trauma care. If Blue Cross muscled Grady into accepting lower payments, it could try to do the same thing with other hospitals that provided trauma care under the state employees plan, the legislators feared. A health committee of the legislature went on record decrying the insurance company's "bullying" of providers.

Just as the 2015 legislature was set to consider a mandate that Blue Cross must cover state-employee health plan enrollees for any bills incurred for trauma care at Grady and the four other Level 1 trauma centers in the state, Blue Cross gave up the fight. Both the state's largest public hospital and the state's largest insurer were conciliatory after the settlement, but the length of the dispute and the public outcry was indicative of how the marketplace was fracturing in the new era of health reform. The issue about how to pay for trauma was front and center, at least for a while anyway.

Trauma as a Revenue Source

In Florida, the haggling over trauma care became much more pitched and wound up in court after HCA, the largest hospital company in the country, decided it wanted to get in the business.

In 2009 HCA revealed plans to open twenty new trauma centers nationwide, more than half of them in Texas and Florida. Most of them were to be in suburban communities, but still within the traditional service area of large public hospitals that were already providing high-level trauma care.

Florida's largest public hospitals—Jackson Memorial in Miami, Tampa General, and Shands Jacksonville Medical Center, among others—balked at the plans. They asked the state to prevent the new centers from opening because their presence would reduce the number of insured patients the larger Level 1 centers needed to stay solvent. The state declined.

The existing trauma centers argued that there was no pressing need for additional trauma centers in most areas of the state where they were being proposed. Moreover, the existing centers needed the volume of patients they were already treating to stay proficient at providing the service. Allowing newer centers to siphon off trauma patients, especially blunt trauma patients, would not only harm the existing centers financially, it would mean competing for the limited number of neurosurgeons, trauma anesthesiologists, and other specialists needed to staff them.

One of the largest, the University of Florida Health Shands Hospital in Gainesville, predicted it would lose about a third of its 2,500 yearly trauma patients if the state allowed the nearby Ocala Regional Medical Center to set up a trauma unit. In Jacksonville, Shands Hospital warned that local taxpayers would have to pick up more of the tab for unpaid trauma services—estimated at about $3 million yearly—if the state allowed the suburban Orange Park Medical Center to get into the trauma business.

Jackson Memorial's Ryder Trauma Center in Miami, the largest in the state, took a $3 million hit in 2012 after Florida okayed Kendall Regional Hospital's request to open a new Level 2 center. Jackson officials estimated at the time that Kendall could siphon away as many as half of its paying patients.

But that argument got nowhere. Indeed, in 2015 the state gave provisional status to another HCA-owned hospital in Miami-Dade County to open a Level 2 center, this one at Aventura Hospital and Medical Center.

At the same time, the state denied an application to open a trauma center at Jackson South Community Hospital, which is owned and operated by the same public entity that owns Jackson Memorial. In the space of four years then, Miami-Dade went from one trauma center to three—two of which were owned by HCA.

Several other Florida cases about trauma services were brought before administrative law judges and appeals courts until 2014 when most of them were settled. The additional trauma centers survived, although it is hard to gauge the real impact more competition in the trauma market has had in Florida—in lives or costs.

But, as a result of the litigation and media inquiries into the dispute, we know more now about one of the motivating factors for reactivating interest in trauma care. The HCA hospitals that sought to provide it had to file information about their charges with the Florida Agency for Health Care Administration.

One of the charges that stood out was something called a "trauma activation fee," which was essentially an automatic fee that is imposed by the hospital to cover a portion of the overhead costs for providing the service. Trauma activation fees, also called trauma resources fees, are not unprecedented. Public hospitals with trauma units charge them too, usually $3,000 to $8,000. The fees are often covered by the patient's insurance plan and can be waived if the patient has no insurance. In some cases, they could be incurred even if the hospital had only stabilized the patient and moved the case to a more advanced trauma facility.

What stood out about the trauma activation fees at these new centers was the high charges some of them imposed.

One HCA hospital, Lawnwood Regional Medical Center in Fort Pierce, Florida, charged, on average, a $29,000 activation fee. Orange Park Medical Center, just south of Jacksonville, averaged $20,000 in activation fee charges. The *Tampa Bay Times* found another Florida HCA hospital charged a few patients $32,000 in trauma activation fees.

More troubling was the prospect that the new trauma centers might be motivated to take in the well-insured blunt trauma victims while stabilizing and transferring the "penetrating" (gunshot wounds, stabbing) victims.

A new era of trauma care has clearly come to Florida. As high trauma activation fees and better coverage for blunt trauma victims becomes more widespread, the trend is expected to take off in other states.

With history as an example of how the marketplace adapts to such changes, it won't be hard to find the hospitals—and patients—left behind.

A $30,000 FEE TO GO TO A TRAUMA CENTER? HOW DID THAT HAPPEN?

If hospital charges seem arbitrary and unreasonable at times, that's because they are. There is no real, predetermined charge for most medical services delivered by a hospital. Instead the charges are based on what hospitals believe insurance companies that cover patients will pay.

The National Uniform Billing Committee of the American Hospital Association plays a major role in determining the legitimacy of the process. If the AHA's committee signs off on the need for certain fees and charges, there is a much better chance that insurance underwriters and Medicare will agree to pay them—or at least agree that hospitals are justified in seeking them. The committee doesn't stipulate what the charge should be. That's up to hospitals and insurance companies to negotiate.

In 2002, when the concept of trauma response fees was first introduced around the country, Connie J.

Porter petitioned the AHA's billing committee to sign off on them. Porter, a registered nurse with an MBA in health administration, is an expert in trauma care. She ran two Level 1 trauma centers in Oregon and was once the state's trauma systems manager.

In an April 2014 *Tampa Bay Times* opinion piece, she explained the intent of the fees. Trauma centers incur significant extra costs because they are usually surgical training centers, and they need expensive diagnostic and surgical equipment and specialists nearby when a trauma patient comes through the door.

Her reasoning prevailed. And with the committee's approval, trauma centers around the country started billing separate trauma activation (or trauma response) fees. Initially, many of them charged $1,500 to $2,000. Now they routinely bill insurance companies of covered patients $3,000 to $6,000. (Almost all of them claim to waive the fees for uninsured trauma patients.)

But in Florida, where for-profit hospitals have decided to get into the trauma business in recent years, these fees can go beyond $30,000, the *Times* reported.

Porter told the newspaper she never imagined her work justifying the fees would become "a back-door way for some hospitals to profiteer."

Florida's recent expansion of trauma centers in for-profit hospitals around the state "threatens to dismantle [the] entire trauma system and undermine a vital pipeline for training surgeons," she wrote. "Floridians need to understand the consequences of such high-profit trauma care and put a stop to it."

So far the state has declined to get involved.

PART III
MARKET PLACES

They are two of our nation's most recognizable public hospitals, but they now stand silent and dark behind eight-foot-tall chain link fences.

Notices posted on the padlocked front doors and emergency room entrances warn the homeless not to seek shelter inside.

On their best days they represented how the country provided compassionate and high-quality care for its poorest and most vulnerable citizens. On their worst days, they were rife with corruption and dangerous to the patients. Now their edifices—one a Depression-era art deco structure with a skybound center tower, the other a World War I–era beaux arts bulwark that occupies two city blocks—are orphans, unwanted in the commercial real estate market and replaced in the health care market by newer hospitals nearby.

Charity of New Orleans and County in Chicago are iconic names in public health history in this country. Within their sprawling wards, tens of thousands of doctors and nurses were trained by taking care of millions of poor and unwanted-anywhere-else patients. For decades, both were vital to the cities they served, even though both—like so many other public hospitals around the country—had serious quality-of-care issues and, at times, seemed almost ungovernable.

Yet the stories connected to Charity's ultimate demise and County's radical transformation represent how public hospitals have adapted to a changing marketplace and the exigencies of local politics in order to survive.

Their legacies raise questions too, about the long-standing commitments of local and state governments to their charitable missions. That pact, going back more than a century in many big cities, was always relatively simple: If you were poor and couldn't afford to get health care anywhere else, you could at least go to Charity or County or the dozens of other large urban hospitals like them to get the care you need.

The distinctively different approaches taken in New Orleans and Chicago are being tried at large public hospitals around the country as these hospitals of last resort for the poor and uninsured seek, anew, to find their place in the nation's $3 trillion health care economy.

Shutting down old, antiquated facilities and starting over may work in some cities—mostly those with a stable tax base that helps secure operations and improvements—while others have to work with what they've got, which often isn't much in the way of local and state support.

The hospitals in this last category are, as a result, the most vulnerable to the whims of local and state politicians and the changing currents of the marketplace.

Atlanta's Grady Memorial Hospital, for instance, continues to struggle in face of local and state political leaders who show little interest in helping it secure its 125-year-old mission to serve the poor and uninsured.

On the other hand, in 2015 Parkland Memorial Hospital in Dallas replaced its aging institution—the place where John F. Kennedy was pronounced dead when he was assassinated—after local voters agreed to put up more than half of the financing for a new $1.3 billion state-of-the-art medical center.

In a nation that still hasn't decided whether health care is a right of citizenship or an earned privilege, this is what public hospitals have always done: they adapt and work with what they are given.

It's important to remember that even after the latest and most ambitious effort in fifty years to provide Americans with affordable health insurance, as much as 15 percent of the population remains without it during any twelve-month period. Most of the uninsured remain in the South where state officials—like those in Georgia, Florida, Texas, and Louisiana—have purposely left behind millions of low-wage workers and the public hospitals that care for them.

Whether that will change, now that the law has survived major legal challenges, seems mostly a question of local and state politics rather than national health policy. In this way, Charity Hospital in New Orleans and County in Chicago symbolize the different approaches to how local government provides and pays for care for the poor.

Indeed, one was literally abandoned after a natural disaster so that it could be replaced. The other more wisely was replaced before it became a disaster.

11

ORPHANS

Charity's Story

Mosquito-borne yellow fever was a scourge of American port cities for decades in the 1700s and 1800s, with New Orleans being the hardest hit. The city endured a series of deadly epidemics every fifteen to twenty years. Mortality reached into thousands during several of the worst outbreaks. Through all of them, the refuge in the public health storm was Charity Hospital, which in 1905—the last epidemic year—was able to contain the death toll to fewer than five hundred. (Among the dead, the New Orleans archbishop, who was said to have contracted the disease from mosquitoes hatched from larvae in the St. Louis Cathedral holy water font.)

An order of Roman Catholic religious women had founded the original Charity in New Orleans in 1736. Along with New York City's Bellevue Hospital, which opened a month earlier, it was the oldest public hospital in the country.

Amazingly, the founding Sisters of Charity stayed involved with the city and ran several replacement hospitals well into the middle of the last century. In fact, the sisters formed an alliance with Governor Huey Long, the city and Franklin D. Roosevelt's New Deal–era public-works agencies and got federal money in 1938 to build the massive public hospital (which at one time had 2,700 beds) that now sits vacant on Tulane Avenue.

Following rapid changes in the health care marketplace after the passage of Medicare and Medicaid, Charity's operations were ceded to the state in 1970. About this same time, the hospital was hit by a series of scandals.

In the mid-1970s, dozens of employees were fired for running prostitution rings and drugs within the hospital's wards. Others were caught stealing food and medical equipment. It became the hospital of last resort for the poor in New Orleans. And for people with money and insurance who got sick, it was the last place they wanted to be.

Charity also had periods when the care it provided was unquestionably second-rate. The defense most often mounted by its advocates was that the competing New Orleans hospitals had no commitment to the poor. Thus Charity, they explained, was forced to treat its overwhelmingly poor clientele quickly, with a baseline level of quality, so that it could serve the constantly increasing demand.

It continued to operate under state control until 1997 when it was absorbed into the LSU Health Sciences system, the state university system that operated about a dozen hospitals in Louisiana at the time, including another one in New Orleans a few blocks away from Charity.

The 2005 decision to close it was a body blow to Charity, much worse than what Katrina did to it.

Despite having the sickest and poorest patients, Charity actually recorded the fewest deaths (eight) of all the flooded hospitals and health care institutions during the storm and its aftermath. (More than 150 patients died at hospitals citywide.)

Charity's medical and nursing staff assumed they would return to work as soon as disaster-recovery officials cleared the old hospital to reopen its doors. Katrina's flood waters had damaged only the basement level of Charity. After the storm, a 200-person team of military and medical personnel brought a 600-kilowatt generator and pumped the water out within a few days.

Their efforts didn't stop there. The entire hospital was swept clean—some said cleaner than it had been before the storm—and "within weeks," according to Lieutenant General Russel

Honoré, who commanded the Katrina task force, Charity would be ready to start receiving patients again.

But it was not to be. Louisiana state government officials had different plans.

Charity had been an unwanted stepchild for years in the fractured marriage among state health officials, LSU, and the city of New Orleans. The state saw it as a money pit and thought it could provide health care for the poor without it.

With millions in federal disaster assistance aid flowing to the city and state—money that went to health care services, rehabilitation and relocation, emergency preparedness, neighborhood development, and other categories that were largely determined by state and local officials—the opportunity to close Charity for good and build a new public hospital largely with the money of federal taxpayers was too much to pass up.

It took a decade and a contentious eminent domain fight with city residents who were pushed out of nearby neighborhoods after Katrina, but, finally, a new $1.1 billion hospital to replace Charity opened in August 2015. The new hospital is owned by the state of Louisiana and called University Medical Center.

Developing it and the area around it was assisted with a healthy dose of disaster relief funds courtesy of US taxpayers. That money included funds to open a network of neighborhood outpatient clinics that are administratively tied to the new medical center—a network that Charity never really had.

And with it, what was once white-hot opposition to the new hospital appears to have evaporated.

It's a done deal now, New Orleans residents seem to have concluded. Like other city neighborhoods touched by Katrina, the surrounding area still has swaths of undeveloped land. It didn't have to be that way, the opponents say. Charity was ready to be reopened and could have been modernized for much less cost. And the displaced residents of the neighborhood could have returned and rebuilt their lives.

Still, most are hopeful that the new University Medical Center will, like the old Charity, become the primary safety-net hospital in what remains an urban region with significant poverty.

The new hospital has many of the things Charity didn't—large, private rooms big enough to accommodate families of patients who want to stay overnight, a rehabilitation services wing, a radiology department within the emergency room, and the state-of-the-art equipment Charity would love to have had but could never quite get the state to pay for when it was in business.

Moreover, the University Medical Center will share several clinical programs with other hospitals nearby, including the Veterans Affairs hospital. Care will be better coordinated, the state promises. The new hospital will take its place as a part of a dynamic, new medical research and clinical care district for the city.

The approach taken in Louisiana is not unlike that followed by many other states, as state governments and their state-financed medical schools assume control of what were once city-owned and city-operated public hospitals. If there is a strong relationship between the medical school staff and hospital administration—including offering profitable medical specialty services, such as cardiac surgery and orthopedics—the public hospital should be able to attract more Medicare and privately insured patients.

Yet catering to private-pay patients is exactly what worries some health care advocates in New Orleans. They fear the high cost of the new hospital will force LSU and the state to eschew indigent patients and those covered by Louisiana's notoriously stingy Medicaid program.

Nor are they encouraged by former Governor Bobby Jindal's efforts over the years to turn over a number of Louisiana's state-owned public hospitals to nonprofit hospital corporations. Indeed, the replacement hospital for Charity is being leased to Children's Hospital and Medical Center, which also operates the private Touro Infirmary, where the poor and uninsured will be sent to deliver babies, since the new medical center has no obstetric services.

Jindal's decision to get the state out of the public hospital business was based in part on the federal government's adjustment to what it pays for Medicaid costs in Louisiana.

After the storm recovery, the Centers for Medicare & Medicaid Services (CMS) said the state would have to put up more for its share of the Medicaid partnership. Rather than lower reimbursement rates for doctors to pay the state's additional costs—which is how most states try to save on Medicaid costs—Jindal directed state health officials to privatize the LSU hospitals.

Jindal—at the time, a Republican running for president—also steadfastly refused to expand Medicaid coverage as envisioned by the ACA to cover more of the working poor who can't afford insurance even with government subsidies. Despite the fact that the federal government would pay 100 percent of the costs through 2016, and no less than 90 percent after that, Jindal's actions left more than 225,000 residents without insurance. His successor, John Bel Edwards, a Democrat elected in November 2015, has pledged to move quickly to expand Medicaid in Louisiana

THE SOUTH AND MEDICAID

Of all the states of the South that made up the old Confederacy, only Arkansas has elected to expand Medicaid under the provisions of the Affordable Care Act of 2010. (And Arkansas was granted permission to create a one-of-a-kind Medicaid plan that allows it to use the money it receives from Washington as a subsidy for new Medicaid enrollees to purchase private insurance.)

The other ten states of the Old South—South Carolina, Mississippi, Alabama, Georgia, Florida, Tennessee, Virginia, North Carolina, Louisiana, and Texas—have all refused to go beyond their current income eligibility levels for residents to qualify for Medicaid. Those strict standards limit Medicaid almost exclusively to the disabled, pregnant women, and young children in low-income families.

Therefore, most adults, regardless of their income, are not eligible for Medicaid. Three of those states, Texas, Florida, and Georgia, now have the highest percentage of uninsured residents in the country and are home to about half of the nation's uninsured residents.

While these states resist joining the new program, they are collectively losing billions of dollars a year in federal funds. In Georgia's case, $9 million a day, which is money that public hospitals serving large numbers of Medicaid and uninsured patients could desperately use.

The South isn't alone in resisting Medicaid expansion. But among the seventeen states and the District of Columbia that the Census Bureau defines as the South—a map that stretches from Texas and Oklahoma east to Maryland and Delaware—eleven of them have refused to go along.

Seven of the twelve states defined as Midwest have similarly refused.

The other states that had not agreed to Medicaid expansion, as of mid-2015, were Oklahoma, Kansas, Missouri, Nebraska, South Dakota, Wyoming, Idaho, Wisconsin, and Maine.

Most experts believe that, as the ACA becomes more accepted, all the states will eventually sign on to the Medicaid expansion. (This assumes, of course, that there will not be a full repeal of the law engineered by some new Republican president and supporting Republican majorities in Congress.) A similar dynamic played out in 1965, when Medicaid was first enacted. It took several states years to join the program. The last, Arizona, didn't agree to it until 1982.

Officials at several of the city's other hospitals are also skeptical that the new hospital will handle the load. They are no doubt still smarting from the unexpected closing of Charity and the forced transfer to their wards of the poor and Medicaid population it once served, even though they too received disaster emergency assistance to offset their costs.

A decade after the storm, New Orleans has yet to decide what to do with the old hospital. There have been several ideas put forward such as turning it into condos, making it mixed-use retail and residential space, even renovating it to become a new City Hall. But the real estate market, like the medical marketplace before it, seems to have relegated Charity to an era whose time has passed.

County's Story

Cook County Hospital's history can be traced back to 1832, when the state of Illinois assigned the care of "pauper patients" to county governments. It was about then when the state's largest county began paying for medical care in temporary hospitals and infirmaries and enlisted the help of Rush Medical School in Chicago.

When a cholera epidemic hit in 1849, the city teamed up with Rush to use one of the medical school's buildings as a hospital. After the Civil War, the city and county purchased an unused building that once housed a reform school, and the first "County" general hospital was opened.

It wasn't long before County was rife with political corruption and poor-quality care, so much so that the entire medical staff resigned, leaving ward bosses to run the place for several decades with doctors and staff of their choosing.

By the turn of a new century, political interference with the hospital had begun to decline. A new civil service law required attending physicians to pass an examination before being allowed to practice there. Chicago's best surgeons and physicians began to work at County. In 1916 they demanded, and got, a brand new hospital—a beaux arts wonder that imposed itself on Harrison Drive in the city's Near West Side, equipped with more than two thousand beds. The new County became home to the nation's first blood bank and other medical innovations that attracted nationwide attention.

It also became home to the city's rapidly increasing African-American population and its diverse base of European ethnic immigrants.

Like Charity in New Orleans, County's patient mix had changed by the time Medicare and Medicaid were enacted, and many workers were covered by insurance on the job. It was left mostly with patients who had no means of paying for their care. And it was forced to start closing beds to survive.

The hospital churned both patients and tax dollars with little or no oversight. For most of its existence, County had been run with no strategic plan. And by the mid-1980s, Medicare and privately insured patients—the patients it needed to sustain its mission—were staying away in droves. The quality of care began to suffer.

Frustrated by a lack of follow-up for their patients after they left the hospital, the attending physician staff formed a professional association and recommended the hospital be transformed to a comprehensive, countywide health care network of primary care clinics and smaller neighborhood hospitals.

Their proposal got nowhere.

About this same time, the physicians at County began to document how other Chicago-area hospitals were refusing to accept indigent patients in their emergency rooms, including pregnant women about to deliver, and sending them to County instead. The practice, known as "patient dumping," was thought to be widespread around the country, but County was the first to prove it.

In 1986, Congress passed the Emergency Medical Treatment and Active Labor Act, which requires hospital ERs to screen all patients coming through their ERs and, at a minimum, stabilize those who are deemed to be in serious condition.

The law, known as EMTALA, remains in force. But the old County Hospital in Chicago is long gone—vacant now since 2002—and, as in New Orleans, the replacement hospital bears little resemblance to it.

Architecturally, John H. Stroger, Jr. Hospital of Cook County is about as dull as it can be, in marked contrast to the vacant hospital down the street with its stone symmetrical facade, balconies, and balustrades. You could easily mistake the old County for an art museum in Italy or France. Yet there is still no viable proposal to find a new use for it.

But few Chicagoans would argue that County then was a better hospital than Stroger is now. Nor does there seem to be much debate that the new hospital, which opened in 2002, has in any way lessened its commitment to care for the poor and uninsured.

Over the years, Cook County took the approach of several other large American cities and counties—most notably, and successfully, Denver—in merging the roles of the public hospital with county health departments. The hospital and clinic network Cook County operates is now the third largest public health system in the country, and it very much resembles the proposal made by the hospital's medical staff in 1986.

By combining vital functions, and paying for them with local tax support, it is easier to coordinate primary health services in neighborhood clinics with the acute-care services at a large hub hospital and one or more smaller community hospitals. Poor and uninsured patients needing health care no longer need rely exclusively on the big public hospital in town.

But the single most important development in securing a brighter future for the new county hospital came more recently with the state's decision to embrace Medicaid expansion under the ACA. Not only did the Illinois state government agree quickly to the expansion, it requested a waiver from federal officials to allow Cook County and Chicago to enroll newly eligible Medicaid patients a year earlier than the rest of the country.

That move allowed County officials to do something innovative among large public hospital systems around the country. They created something called CountyCare —an HMO-type insurance plan that provides a medical home for newly enrolled Medicaid patients for a flat, fixed yearly fee for all the services they may need.

County was able to pull this off because of its own network of primary care clinics in the city and county, as well as its own community hospitals. Moreover, the Medicaid program is now connected to sixteen federally qualified primary health care centers that get operating subsidies from the federal government to treat low-income patients.

In many cities these vital players in health care for the poor have been inexplicably left to operate independently from the public hospitals that serve the same communities. By teaming up with CountyCare, the federal health centers and the local public hospital system have an incentive now to coordinate better care for the Medicaid population they serve.

Richard Romanowski, a self-employed musician in Chicago, is one of the enrollees in CountyCare. Unable to afford insurance of his own, and making too much to qualify for Medicaid prior to the expansion, Romanowski rarely went to the doctor, despite being diagnosed with diabetes and showing obvious symptoms of high blood pressure and heart disease.

Like others in his sixties without insurance, Romanowski told Chicago public television station, WTTW in 2014 that he was trying to wait out the clock until he was old enough for Medicare to get the help he needed. But when CountyCare became available to him at age sixty-two, he quickly enrolled. Now he is able to get consistent monitoring and medications through the new county-run program. He feels better, even though his physician at the center insists he stay away from the sodas and ice cream treats that he loves.

Better still, the risk of Richard Romanowski being rushed to County's emergency room because of a stroke or heart attack or other complications of diabetes has been significantly reduced. That's a win for him and for Cook County taxpayers.

Whether state and local officials in other parts of the country ever come to understand this concept may be the key to the future of America's public hospitals.

12

HOPE AND REALITY

The Mercy Care clinic on Decatur Street is what's left of the legacy of the four Sisters of Mercy who came to Atlanta with only their faith and fifty cents to open St. Joseph's, the city's first real hospital in 1880.

The pioneering nuns are gone, of course, and their religious order recently got out of the hospital business in Atlanta. The latest iteration of the hospital they founded is in an area dubbed "Pill Hill" in Atlanta's northern suburb of Sandy Springs, where two other hospitals and numerous physician office buildings surround it. It is owned and operated now by Emory Healthcare, Atlanta's largest health system. Ironically, as of mid-2015, only four religious women remain at work at Emory–St. Joseph's Hospital.

The foundation that runs Mercy Care was created in 1978 when St. Joseph's moved to the suburbs, and the religious order wanted to make certain that its mission of caring for the poor in the inner city was not abandoned. Indeed, Mercy Care has become the largest provider of health services to the city's large homeless population, and it plays an essential role in seeing to it that poor people with HIV/AIDs and behavioral health conditions get the care they need.

Ninety percent of Mercy Care's patients have no insurance whatsoever.

In this way, its mission is similar to that of Grady Memorial Hospital, Atlanta's giant public hospital across Interstate 75/85 from the largest Mercy Care clinic: to offer health services to anyone who needs them, regardless of ability to pay. It harkens to a similar time in the 1880s when St. Joseph's, a faith-filled dream of the Sisters of Mercy, and Henry W. Grady Memorial Hospital, a civic enterprise named after the man who championed it from an editor's pulpit, helped Atlanta awaken to the health care needs of the poor.

Mercy Care employs a handful of primary care doctors and nurse practitioners at its five Atlanta clinics. They are assisted by volunteer physicians who provide a range of services at the clinics, in mobile vans, and several hours a week at Atlanta's churches, homeless shelters, and other locations. The clinics get about $4 million annually from the federal government to provide care to Atlanta's "underserved" population. They get nothing directly from state or local governments.

Yet Mercy Care and Grady, which have existed in the same community for more than thirty-five years, rarely have worked together. Doctors at the Mercy Care clinic could not admit patients to Grady when they needed to be hospitalized. And when Grady discharged its indigent patients, it had no way of getting medical records and other clinical information to the nonprofit clinic if the patient needed follow-up care.

That changed in 2015 when Grady's administrators and local public health advocates decided, finally, that it would be better to coordinate care—rather than duplicate services and compete—in a state and region that provides comparatively little in the way of public financing for indigent care services.

Grady and Mercy Care exchange patients, medical records, and physicians now. They can coordinate care in ways designed to ensure their indigent and low-income patients stay healthy and out of the hospital.

What seems like an obvious step toward better public health now could not have been accomplished a few short years ago. And it may not come to full fruition if state officials continue to obstruct modest efforts to expand Medicaid services to the poor.

Traditionally, federally subsidized community health centers like Mercy Care—and five similar clinics operated by other nonprofit groups in Fulton and DeKalb counties—fiercely guarded their independent, nonprofit status. They wanted nothing to do with the politics and administration of public hospitals like Grady. And, as in Grady's case, they were probably smart to keep their distance. Until recently, Grady was a mess.

But the onetime wreck of a public hospital has made a huge turnaround in recent years, which makes the state of Georgia's resistance toward helping it coordinate health care to the working poor yet another example of a missed opportunity.

Saving Grady

In 2008 the hospital was gushing red ink. It owed the two medical schools that provided its medical staff—Emory University and the Morehouse School of Medicine—more than $60 million. Pharmaceutical companies and vendors were complaining of late payments or no payment at all. And there was constant speculation within the staff that Grady would not meet the next payroll.

The Fulton-DeKalb Hospital Authority, which owned and operated Grady, had swept through four chief executive officers in just five years. It had just fired its fourth and installed the chairwoman of the authority, a state representative, as the hospital's latest CEO. Despite no hospital administration experience—she was an attorney in a small practice by herself—the new CEO was rewarded with the same $600,000 yearly salary as the man who preceded her.

Grady had been through turmoil like this before, but nothing quite as bad.

In the early 1990s, the authority issued bonds for a much-needed renovation and expansion of Grady. The price tag was more than $300 million, at the time the largest public-works project in the history of the state.

It didn't go well.

The project was beset with cost overruns and charges of political interference. White-owned companies on the job were reported to be paid above their contract rate in order to give work to minority subcontractors so they would be in compliance with Fulton County's minority contracting rules. The arrangement caused a major fallout between the hospital authority that was paying the bills and the Fulton County Commission, which was insisting on minority participation.

Several floors in one tower of the hospital that were supposed to be renovated didn't get finished. Because of the overruns, the hospital came up 269 beds short of its planned capacity.

A few years after that, the hospital was swimming in debt again. Governor Roy Barnes, a Democrat, found a way to channel $40 million in additional Medicaid funding from the state to bail out Grady. In return, the hospital promised to do a better job of collecting debt and overseeing expenses.

Grady instituted some cost-savings programs and cleaned up its contract-oversight process. But the medical schools did not force timely payment of what they were owed, and the hospital continued to accumulate a growing mountain of debt.

Furthermore, one of the state's top politicians—State Senate Majority Leader Charles Walker—was caught up in yet another contract scandal at Grady. It involved a $1.5 million deal to provide the hospital with laundry and housecleaning workers through a temporary services company he owned. Walker failed to disclose the public contract and was fined by the state ethics committee. He later was convicted in federal court of tax evasion, theft, and strong-arming Grady administrators into awarding his company the contract.

In 2007, the Grady Hospital Foundation hired a private health care consulting firm to recommend cost-saving measures and other administrative changes to restore financial stability. The hospital authority dismissed most of the recommendations—especially those involving tough decisions about personnel and operations—and ignored others. The effort cost the foundation $2 million. (Interestingly, two years later the new governing board would implement several of the consultant's proposals.)

News reports in the *Atlanta Journal-Constitution* made it clear that Governor Sonny Perdue and the state's new Republican leadership would not move to bail out Grady again, even as it teetered on the brink that same year. "It's unlikely Perdue will ever appreciate Grady's importance," the *Journal-Constitution's* Cynthia Tucker wrote.

It was arguably a shortsighted decision since Grady trains one in every four doctors practicing in the state and provides Georgia's highest level of trauma and neonatal services, its only sickle-cell program, a first-rate burn center, and one of the largest HIV/AIDs clinics in the Southeast—specialty services that are extended to patients from throughout much of the state, not just Atlanta.

Georgia was getting a bargain, considering that it provided almost no direct state funding for Grady's operational expenses. Still, state officials seemed willing to let Grady go down.

Fulton and DeKalb counties, which by contract are required to provide operating subsidies for the hospital, froze their support as well. A taxpayer revolt in Fulton County installed a new Republican county commission chairman in the wake of the Grady renovation fiasco in the late 1990s. And the Republican members of subsequent county commissions wanted nothing to do with sending more money to the hospital.

The numbers tell the story about the decline in local funding. In 1995, Fulton and DeKalb put up about $100 million—75 percent of it coming from Fulton, the state's largest county—toward Grady's $400 million operating budget. This amount was roughly in keeping with the 1984 contract the two counties promised Grady they would appropriate for their share of charges Grady incurred for taking care of the "indigent sick" of Fulton and DeKalb counties.

But in 2005, the two counties were providing Grady about the same amount, even though the hospital's operating budget was then up to $670 million and its load of indigent patients was rapidly increasing.

Yet, Grady survived, not because of any help from the state of Georgia or a renewed commitment to charity care on the part of the two counties that own it. Grady survived because local business leaders understood it was too important to fail.

As the hospital balanced on the edge, the Metro Atlanta Chamber of Commerce and other civic groups assembled a task force that recommended day-to-day management of Grady be taken away from the hospital authority and turned over to a nonprofit management corporation, the way many other public hospitals and health systems have transformed themselves around the country over the last thirty years.

The head of the task force, former Georgia-Pacific CEO Pete Correll, spent months lobbying elected leaders at the state and local level. By turning Grady over to be run by an independent board—not political appointees—the hospital stood a good chance of restoring faith with the community, he said. If the hospital could reform its management, Correll promised to work toward raising $200 million in foundation and philanthropic grants so that Grady could modernize equipment and refurbish whole departments of the hospital while it was getting back on its financial feet.

His toughest job was in persuading black leaders in the two counties that it was a good plan and did not amount to "a white takeover" of Grady—a phrase commonly used to deride the plan. He concentrated his lobbying efforts on the powerful ministerial community in Atlanta that had rallied in the past against major reductions in Grady's staff. Just a few years earlier, the ministers also fought hard against proposals that some of Grady's low-income patients pay small, out-of-pocket costs for prescription drugs. He enlisted the help of Michael Russell, CEO of H. J. Russell & Co., one of the largest black-owned construction companies in the country. (The firm was founded by his father, Herman J. Russell.)

There was racial history to overcome as well. Many could still remember when the new hospital was built in 1958. Like the segregated hospitals that preceded it, they continued to call the new hospital "the Gradys," because it was designed with segregated wings.

That changed with the Civil Rights Act and the enactment of Medicare and Medicaid in the 1960s. And by the 1990s, the hospital's administration and the two-county authority that ran it was heavily dominated by African-Americans. The ministers and other black leaders in the region worried that the Chamber of Commerce folks now pushing the new governance plan would abandon Grady's historic mission, or perhaps sell the hospital to a for-profit company.

Despite their misgivings, black leaders and the county commissions signed off on the plan. (The firing of the last administrator and the hiring of the authority chairwoman to run the hospital in early 2008 proved to be the last straw.)

The authority still owned the hospital, but it agreed that a new governing board, headed by Correll, would run it. A new administrator was hired to whip it into shape—the kind of "change agent" businesspeople like, but public employees loathe and fear.

One story has it that the new boss, who was strolling the hallways one night by himself, came upon a nurses' station and found only one nurse on duty. To make matters worse, she was asleep on the job. The boss affixed a sticky note to the nurse's hospital ID while she slept. "You're fired," the note said. "Report to Human Resources when you wake up." (The story is probably urban hospital legend, but it is indicative that Grady was indeed entering a new era.)

Public Hospitals and Questions of Care

It is also the kind of story you routinely hear about public hospitals, which rightly or wrongly, have a reputation as operating in the highly competitive health care sector with all the customer service traits of a department of motor vehicles office.

That too is changing, but truth be told, nearly every public hospital in the country has had similar problems with mismanagement, political interference, and quality of care.

The scandals range from financial improprieties to horrific treatment of the very patients they were chartered to help.

In 2004, a surveillance camera captured a hospital maintenance worker nonchalantly mopping the floor around a patient who had fallen and was unresponsive in a corridor outside the emergency room at the Martin Luther King/Charles Drew Medical Center in Los Angeles.

The patient left unattended on the floor was a forty-three-year-old mother of three, who later died. A yearlong investigation by the *Los Angeles Times* determined the county-run facility had repeatedly harmed or killed patients and that several departments were rife with incompetence, infighting, and, sometimes, criminality.

Like defenders of other public hospitals that have run into trouble over the years, advocates for King/Drew said the problem was inadequate public funding. Indeed, that was the persistent claim made by critics of the Grady management change. The state and local governments simply needed to give Grady more money for operating expenses, and things would be fine, they said.

But how much money public hospitals get from government coffers—while obviously essential to their mission—is probably less important than how effectively the money is spent. More importantly, by demonstrating the money is being spent wisely, public hospitals can make a better case for getting more of it when they need it.

In comparison to other, similar-sized public hospitals in LA County, King/Drew handled fewer patients and spent much more on its staff, with high rates of absenteeism and little supervision, the *Times* reported. There was no coordination of care, and the hospital was top-heavy with highly paid administrators.

With its quality-of-care issues so widespread, Los Angeles County shut down the hospital as an acute-care facility after the federal government refused to authorize it to take any more Medicare and Medicaid patients in 2007. Fortunately, the county's large public hospital network seemed to be able to absorb the influx of former King/Drew patients. The hospital reopened—on a much smaller scale and with more supervision—in 2015. But thanks to the new health care law, the county does not expect it to handle nearly as many poor patients as it did when it ran into trouble.

At Parkland Memorial Hospital in Dallas, the quality of care was serious enough in 2011 that the Centers for Medicare & Medicaid Services intervened. Rather than stop paying for care, like it did in Los Angeles, CMS took a different route with the much bigger Texas hospital. It sent independent overseers to Dallas to help get the place in compliance again. (Alvarez & Marsal Healthcare Industry Group, the consulting firm that was hired, then fired at Grady in 2007, was chosen to whip Parkland back in shape.)

It should be noted that the problems at Parkland were not as desperate as in Los Angeles. Still, they involved everything from discharge planning—several psychiatric patients had died shortly after leaving the hospital—to infection control, staff training, and monitoring of nurses and physicians.

Many of the quality-of-care issues could be traced not to lack of funding, but to the uneasy relationship Parkland had at the time with the University of Texas Southwestern Medical School, which staffs the hospital.

Like most other public hospitals with medical school affiliations, the hospital does not actually employ the medical school doctors who see patients there. The *Dallas Morning News* found in 2013 that many of the UTSW faculty members left their resident doctors-in-training unsupervised at Parkland and instead concentrated their clinical attention on privately insured patients at other hospitals in Dallas that are wholly owned and run by UTSW.

This is a common complaint among public hospital administrators.

In many large cities, the medical schools that staff public hospitals have their own highly profitable hospitals and clinics elsewhere in the community. Privately insured patients of medical school faculty are much more likely to be treated at those facilities rather than at the public hospital—leading to sometimes tense relationships.

In Atlanta, by way of comparison, the Emory University School of Medicine's highest-profile services—cardiovascular surgery and cardiology, transplant medicine, cancer research and clinical care—are all housed at the University Hospital and medical buildings on Emory's suburban Druid Hills campus, six miles away. Those services are also available at Grady, but on a more limited scale. And the patients who use them there are more likely to be indigent or covered by Medicaid.

In Dallas, Parkland's failure to exercise control over the clinical care services provided by UTSW was a direct contributor to inadequate patient care, according to the newspaper and other subsequent investigations of problems at the hospital.

Thanks to intensive federal oversight, changes in hospital administration, and a better relationship with UTSW, Parkland seems to have survived its crisis years. Indeed, in August of 2015, the sixty-year-old hospital (whose emergency room entrance became familiar to Americans when the assassinated President John F. Kennedy was rushed there on November 22,

1963) was replaced by a $1.3 billion state-of-the-art hospital across the street.

Dallas taxpayers put up more than half of that amount in a bond issue, which seems to indicate they have confidence that Parkland is on the right track. And Parkland's administrators are clearly betting on being able to compete in the Dallas marketplace, even if Texas—like many other Southern states—has decided not to expand Medicaid coverage, as envisioned in the new health care reform law, to hundreds of thousands of low-income residents.

The Politics of Public Hospitals

Not long after Rick Scott was elected governor of Florida in 2010, all the public hospitals in the state were ordered to do something unusual. Scott, a former chief executive of the for-profit HCA chain of hospitals, and fellow Republicans in the state legislature wanted to see if there might be a market for selling off or leasing some of the Sunshine State's public hospitals to for-profit or nonprofit competitors.

The concept of leasing a public hospital to a for-profit company is not unprecedented. Conservatives have long claimed that investor-owned institutions could run public hospitals more efficiently and make them more appealing to insured patients.

Thirty years earlier, the state of Kentucky cut a deal with Humana, then a huge hospital company based in Louisville, to manage the new University of Louisville Hospital, the replacement for the old Louisville General Hospital. The company named the facility Humana Hospital-University, bolstering the image it was trying to cultivate at the time as providing not just clinical care, but cutting-edge research.

The company and the state eventually parted ways. Humana, concluding there was more money to be made selling insurance, decided to get out of the hospital business. And the state eventually decided a nonprofit consortium should run University Hospital.

More recently, in 2010, Vanguard Health Systems, a Nashville-based investor-owned company that operated hospitals and nursing homes, purchased the Detroit Medical Center's eight hospitals. The price was a relatively paltry $364 million. But at that time, the Detroit system was $417 million in debt. The state of Michigan had balked at providing additional funding for the Detroit hospitals, and local nonprofit hospitals had no interest in the public facilities. Vanguard pledged to sink $850 million in capital improvements during the first five years of its ownership of DMC—much of it to increase the size of Detroit Receiving Hospital, the system's best-known facility.

The deal with Vanguard, now owned by Tenet Healthcare, appears to have stabilized the DMC financial picture.

Perhaps this is what Florida legislators had in mind when a private equity firm made a pitch, which was subsequently withdrawn, to acquire Jackson Memorial, Florida's largest public hospital, in Miami.

Ostensibly the 2012 law that Florida enacted was simply to clarify state statutes that some believed made selling or leasing public institutions to private buyers illegal. But it went a step further than that. It ordered all the public hospitals in the state to "commence an evaluation of the possible benefits" to the community if a buyer could be found. The evaluations were to be made public to local and state government officials.

The law even included provisions for how the money from any potential sales should be distributed. (Half of it would go to a health care economic-development trust fund to promote job creation in the health care sector.)

Interestingly, the law didn't require the hospitals to study any potential risks to a sale, although most of the hospitals that complied with the law were quick to point those out.

Nor did it seem to be all that interested in the current

economic impact of the existing hospitals. And, to date, it hasn't resulted in any of the government-owned hospitals being sold, since many of them operate on tight revenue-over-expenses margins that require substantial philanthropic and local tax support to stay in business.

Nonetheless, the state's attitude toward public hospitals seemed clear: Before you come asking for more money from state or local taxpayers, we want to know if we can unload you first.

This wasn't good news for Jackson Memorial Hospital and its Miami-Dade County system of public hospitals and clinics. The health system was pushing upwards of $500 million of bad debt, charity care, and losses from caring for patients in Florida's Medicaid program.

The new CEO at Jackson, Carlos A. Migoya, a former banker and Miami city manager, had engineered a remarkable turnaround, taking it from an $82 million loss in 2010 to an $8 million surplus in 2011. But Jackson Memorial clearly was—and remains—heavily reliant on sales and property taxes the state authorizes local counties to collect for public hospital operations.

Moreover, after the Supreme Court ruling in 2012 that allowed states to opt out of Medicaid expansion, Scott and the Republican legislature took a hard stand for just that—denying insurance to an estimated 800,000 people who would have qualified for it if they lived in Michigan, New York, California, or one of the thirty states that have enacted Medicaid expansion. That one decision continues to put the most financial pressure on the state's public hospitals, which could have seen substantial new revenue, and a corresponding reduction in charity care, had Florida agreed to it instead of rejecting it.

THE REPUBLICAN ALTERNATIVES
TO MEDICAID EXPANSION

It's often easy to understand what many of the Republican governors in the Southern states are against—Medicaid expansion, like the kind called for in the Affordable Care Act. They complain, often and loudly, about it all the time. But exactly what they propose as an alternative is a little harder to decipher. Nor has there been any significant movement in Congress to enact alternatives to the program.

The year after the ACA was passed in Congress, the Republican Governor's Association declared it wanted more flexibility for states to determine how best to provide health care coverage for the poor. Rather than endorsing the ACA's approach, which calls for Medicaid to cover individuals and families making up to 135 percent of the federal poverty level, most Republican governors want to greatly loosen the reins the federal government demands on how Medicaid works.

Nevertheless, New Jersey, Ohio, and several other states with Republican governors have accepted the ACA's expansion, which in its first three years is paid for entirely with federal tax dollars. (After that, states start picking up some of the costs, but never more than 10 percent, according to the ACA.)

This fact that the states will eventually have to pick up some share of the cost is at the heart of the opposition now, especially in the South. Governors of these states have declared that expansion of Medicaid is "unaffordable."

The 100 percent federal funding provision expires in 2016, when it begins to be scaled back each year until it reaches a 90 percent floor. The ACA was designed that way because Congress knew the expansion would be expensive as millions of previously uninsured Americans began to enroll in Medicaid and seek medical care they may have been putting off.

Many Republican governors and state legislators simply don't trust the federal government's promise to pay that much of the cost. A budget crisis at the federal level could easily result in states having to bear a much bigger financial burden, the governors say. And in economic recessions, more Americans will turn to Medicaid for coverage, and with medical costs always on the rise, Medicaid will become an even larger burden on state budgets than it already is.

What do they propose instead?

Southern Republican governors, like Georgia's Nathan Deal, want the federal government to provide a yearly fixed amount of funding for Medicaid, in the form of a block grant. They want the money to come with few or no strings attached. The states would be able to set their own eligibility standards and benefit packages for low-income individuals and families. In exchange, the federal government could cap spending on Medicaid, now the largest government health insurance program—bigger even than Medicare.

Among other things, Republican states would like to be able to charge a sliding-scale premium for Medicaid coverage and impose yearly deductibles and out-of-pocket costs. This is how most private insurance plans work. Many of these types of cost-containing provisions the governors call for are either banned by current Medicaid rules or require the federal government to sign off on them. (Arkansas, the lone Republican-led state in the South to accept Medicaid expansion, got permission to set up its state program with some of these provisions.)

Health advocates dislike the block grant approach for the same reason Republicans in statehouses and Congress love it: it usually locks in a fixed amount of spending. Indeed, virtually all of the block grant proposals currently in Congress call for massive reduction in spending on Medicaid, as much as $732 billion at the federal level over the next decade.

The Kaiser Family Foundation, in an independent analysis of then-House Budget Chairman Paul Ryan's block grant proposal, estimated that 14 to 22 million people would need to come off Medicaid by 2022 if states did not supplement funding for the program.

Health advocates worry that when economic hard times happen, both Washington and state capitals would be unlikely to cough up the extra money, which would mean further restricting eligibility, cutting benefits, and crippling the only US program that is supposed to protect low-income Americans.

Perhaps the critical question to ask is this: Will the block grant program be an improvement in getting access to health care for the poor, or is it just a scheme to spend less money on them?

Jackson's stability has been boosted considerably by its strong relationship with the University of Miami School of Medicine, which houses many of its specialty services. Those services include the Miami Transplant Institute, which performs more than 450 organ transplants annually, on the Jackson campus. Not too bad for a hospital that the state seemed interested in selling off for parts just a few years ago.

The connection that large public hospitals have with public

medical schools is worth noting here. When governors, state legislators, and health officials have a stake in securing adequate resources for the state's publicly financed medical schools, they seem to work more cooperatively with the teaching hospitals those schools need. The reverse also seems to be true. Public hospitals that draw staff from private medical schools have a harder time getting the attention of state officials when they are in need. This is an ongoing issue for Grady and helps explain the state's indifference to the Atlanta public hospital.

Still, even with the University of Miami Medical School's partnership, more than half of Jackson's patients are indigent and unable to pay, or Medicaid covers them. Until it gets more Medicare and privately insured patients—or the state has a change of heart about Medicaid expansion—local taxpayers must continue to support it.

Saving Grady, the Sequel

Pete Correll found Grady to be in even worse shape than he had imagined before the takeover in 2008.

At one point, Correll himself had to write a personal check for several million dollars just so the hospital could make its payroll—money that eventually was transferred as a gift to the hospital from him and his wife to improve cardiac care services.

The new board also found that thousands of "Grady cards"—essentially an ID that allowed the holder to get free care at Grady if they had paperwork to show their low-income status—were in the hands of people who never got their income verified. (A few Grady cards had even been provided to the families of elected public officials as a "courtesy.")

The cards were created by the hospital authority years earlier to ensure only Fulton and DeKalb residents got free care at Grady. Indeed, hundreds of indigent patients a year are admitted to Grady, even though they live outside the two counties and Grady has no obligation to serve them. Most of them come from Clayton County in the south metro region—a poor county with a financially troubled public hospital of its own.

The Grady card idea didn't really solve that issue, and it had an unintended side effect. Cardholders showing up at the hospital were rarely quizzed to see if they qualified for Medicaid, Medicare, or private insurance that could have covered the cost of the services.

The new administration did away with Grady cards.

The new governing board also changed the hospital's pension plan for new employees to reverse years of chronic underfunding. And the new CEO made Grady's staff toe a hard workday line, ending a system where they could clock in and out of work via telephone and replacing it with a traditional punch clock. (Hospital administrators had to use the new system as well.)

Even with the turmoil—or perhaps because of it—the money that Correll promised from local business and philanthropic leaders started to flow toward Grady Memorial.

The Robert W. Woodruff Foundation, named after the legendary Atlanta civic leader who ran Coca-Cola for five decades, put up $200 million over four years. Much of that money from the city's largest philanthropy went to improvements in the hospital's information technology system, software for its imaging equipment, renovation of some semiprivate rooms to private rooms—all capital improvements Grady had delayed, some of them for longer than a decade, while it lurched from crisis to crisis.

The Marcus Foundation, the philanthropic arm of Bernie Marcus, cofounder of Atlanta-based Home Depot, stepped up to provide $50 million, most of it toward improvements to Grady's highest-profile services. Marcus money first went to rebuild the hospital's trauma center as well as the stroke and neuroscience center. Both centers, which now bear his name, offer the most advanced specialty services in the state.

Marcus money went as well to reconstruct the rest of Grady's entire emergency department, the hospital's unofficial front door. Nearly three quarters of Grady's admissions come through the emergency department. The emergency department sees more than 115,000 patients a year.

For years, the always-crowded waiting room has looked more like a bus station for sick and injured passengers than a health care facility. When patients finally make it through triage and waiting to be treated in the ER, their families are often left behind because of lack of space in the treatment area.

The new emergency department includes "mini" private rooms that are designed with enough space to allow families to accompany patients while they are treated. The improvements are allowing hospital officials to think that the new facility will actually attract insured patients who need the high-quality emergency care that Grady provides and may no longer be put off by the bus-station atmosphere of its old ER. It will undoubtedly take years to overcome that reputation.

Still, it is important to remember that most of these improvements at Grady and other public hospitals are the result of private funding, not tax dollars from the state or local counties.

Indeed, the state continues to treat Grady as a local hospital that should not be Georgia's problem.

Over the years, Georgia has provided a small amount of funding for some of Grady's specialty services, such as its burn center, which takes in patients from all over north Georgia. The trauma center also gets some money to coordinate with a regional network of first responders and other hospitals.

But there is no mechanism in Georgia, as there is in some other states, to help finance public health and hospital services. The state provides money so that regional districts and counties can offer public health department services, but none of that goes to acute hospital care, and only a relatively small amount goes to basic preventive services such as childhood immunizations and well-baby care. There is state funding for mental health and substance abuse on a regional basis, but, again, very little of that makes its way toward general public hospitals for the operational costs they incur by treating these patients.

Instead, Georgia's public hospitals essentially rely on two major sources of government funding to stay in business: Medicaid reimbursement, mostly limited to low-income pregnant women and children they treat, and local tax dollars to offset the estimated $1.5 billion they lose annually by treating adults with no means of paying their bills.

That's the continuing challenge Grady faces. Unlike the business and philanthropic community in Atlanta, neither state nor local political leaders have stepped up to help the hospital become more financially secure.

Fulton and DeKalb counties have actually reduced funding for the hospital over the past two decades. In 2013 they provided just over $60 million toward Grady's operations. That figure was about 8 percent of the hospital's $764 million operating budget. (By comparison, the 1995 allocation from the two counties amounted to 25 percent of Grady's operating budget.)

To some extent the business community's made-good promise to help out Grady seems to have lulled local officials into justifying a reduction in their contractual responsibilities to the hospital.

Each year during budget deliberations, Fulton County conducts a minidrama of public posturing with the hospital and state officials, arguing, at times, that Grady should be getting more money from the state, or that Grady must do a better job of proving its indigent care costs, or that the state's continuing efforts to restrict the county tax base means Grady will get even less local money next year. And, after that performance, it manages to find money—sometimes a little more, often a little less than the year before—to throw Grady's way.

It is a tiresome exercise, hospital officials acknowledge, but one they must go through even if local funding remains unstable. Grady needs all the help it can get.

At the state level, the disinterest in appropriating money for indigent care isn't directed specifically at Grady. It is mostly an ideological animosity toward the ACA—or as it is always called in Georgia, Obamacare—and more specifically Medicaid. But the implications directly impact Grady, which could significantly reduce its charity load if more of its adult patients were covered by the federal-state program.

Unlike other nonexpansion states where governors and legislative leaders have at least considered the economic benefits of making Medicaid available to low-income, working adults, Georgia's political leadership condemns the concept as too expensive and unworkable. (That leadership includes the state's elected insurance commissioner who proclaimed in 2014 that he would do everything in his power to obstruct the implementation of the ACA in Georgia.)

At the height of the debate in 2013 over expansion, William Custer, a respected health policy and economics expert at Georgia State University, produced a detailed report that showed expanding Medicaid would generate more than 50,000 new jobs in Georgia and $65 billion in new economic activity. Moreover, at a cost of about 1 percent of the state's $20 billion annual budget, expansion would infuse the state with an additional $276 million a year in new tax revenue, Custer reported—probably enough to offset the state's additional spending on the program.

And then there was this assessment based on research published in the *New England Journal of Medicine*: Expansion would save the lives of approximately 1,179 people in Georgia each year, people who would otherwise die because they couldn't afford the health care they need.

State leaders ignored these and other reports from nonpartisan sources about the wisdom of expansion. It was as if they didn't exist.

When asked about them, the governor, insurance commissioner, and legislative leadership dismissed them as made-up numbers and the work of liberal advocacy groups who are out of touch with Georgia voters.

In 2014, fearing the remote possibility that a Democrat might win the governorship that year and decide to expand Medicaid, the general assembly passed a law giving that authority exclusively to itself.

Tax Breaks for Jobs or Spending on the Poor?

The attitude of Georgia's elected leadership toward health care speaks volumes toward the state's priorities.

In the same time frame Grady and public health advocates were clamoring for Medicaid expansion, the state and virtually all its elected leadership, including the mayor of Atlanta, were shuttling back and forth to Washington trying to secure federal funding to dredge the river channel leading to the Port of Savannah.

The port project was essential to Georgia's economic development, the state's leaders—including the governor, US senators, legislative leaders, and the congressional delegation—contended. Without federal money to support the project, vital new shipping business would go to ports elsewhere on the Eastern Seaboard. The state's Republican officials chafed at what they saw as the Obama administration's partisan disinterest in the project.

Yet these same elected officials have consistently rejected the $9 million a day that the ACA could be sending to the state—more than $30 billion over ten years—to expand Medicaid and make health care available to 500,000 to 600,000 residents who now go without it.

Conversely, the state is quick to tout what appears to be a

very successful tax credit scheme that has attracted the television and movie-making business to the Peach State in recent years. For any production company that spends $500,000 or more making a movie or TV show in Georgia, the state offers up to a 30 percent tax credit on spending within the state. And if the company has little or no tax liability in the first place, it can sell its tax credit to another company.

The state doesn't provide specific numbers about how much revenue is lost by the film tax credit scheme, but a good estimate in 2010 was that it amounted to about $140 million yearly. Since then, the film business is busier than ever in Georgia. One recent estimate said it generates about $6 billion in economic impact, most of it coming from nearly 80,000 jobs connected to studio and on-location productions.

Interestingly, the state chooses to proclaim these economic impact projections as gospel, while decrying the Medicaid projections as manufactured by advocacy groups.

The point is not that the state should give up its economic development projects like the Port of Savannah, or do away with the movie-industry tax credits. Now that the harsh impact of the recession is behind it, the state budget is showing healthy surpluses again.

The point is instead about priorities. All evidence indicates the state can more than afford to expand Medicaid and continue its economic development projects too. It simply isn't a priority for state officials to do that. Not now, anyway.

Yet despite the state's indifference, there is still cautious optimism at the 125-year-old hospital.

In 2013, Grady posted a net income of more than $19 million, according to financial documentation it provided to CMS. The CEO and other administrators reported in mid-2015 that it should close its most recent fiscal year with a $12 million to $16 million surplus—quite a different financial picture than what was happening a decade ago when Grady was headed toward a $50 million loss.

But while that bottom line may seem healthy, Grady's operating expenses are north of $750 million annually.

Correll, who will leave Grady's board in 2016, said he hopes to build a reserve fund that could be used in the event of an economic downturn or unexpected expenses in future years. He had a modest goal when the new governing board took over the hospital in 2008, he said.

"Grady will pay all its debts and never get to the crisis point that it was in when it almost had to close," he said. Through a $20 million debt-forgiveness arrangement by Emory, and in its first years under new leadership, Grady finally repaid the two medical schools that had essentially served as its bank during the worst times. "We will make the hard decisions that need to be made before that would happen again," Correll pledged.

The recent courtship between the hospital and the Mercy Care clinic is an example of Grady's search for new ways to care for the poor. It's a part of a much larger plan Grady and other safety-net providers in the Atlanta area have hatched to work around Georgia's refusal to expand Medicaid.

The proposal for Atlanta is modeled after a successful program in Cleveland launched in 2013. MetroHealth Medical Center (Cleveland's version of Grady) teamed up with the city's federally qualified health centers (like Mercy Care) to provide hospital and primary care services to nearly 30,000 Cuyahoga County residents who had been without insurance.

MetroHealth and the primary care clinics persuaded federal and state officials to cover the target population under Medicaid expansion earlier than had been planned in order to see if, by working together, they could better control costs and improve patient health. MetroHealth assumed the financial risk for the experiment, assuring state and federal officials that if total costs were more than what Medicaid provided, it would absorb the expenses. The new program was called MetroHealth Care.

In a July 2015 issue of *Health Affairs*, health policy experts at Case Western Reserve University examined MetroHealth Care's results. Their findings showed that the consortium was able to provide extensive primary care services, as well as acute hospital care, at a cost of about 30 percent below what was budgeted to cover the newly enrolled patients.

Equally important, the study showed that MetroHealth Care significantly improved both the quality of care as well as clinical outcomes for diabetic patients enrolled in the program, compared to a control group of uninsured patients with diabetes. There were improvements in care and outcomes for hypertensive patients as well, the study's authors found.

Uncontrolled diabetes, hypertension, and other chronic conditions are major drivers of indigent care costs at public hospital emergency rooms. Bending the cost-of-care curve on these and other chronic conditions by improving primary care access and treatment, even slightly, would go a long way toward reducing the pressure on safety-net hospitals.

This is why one of the provisions of the ACA is to encourage hospitals and doctors to create accountable care organizations to coordinate services for Medicare and Medicaid patients. The financial incentives within the new law to do so have been driving hospitals to acquire physician practices in the private sector since the passage of the ACA. Now that same trend line is playing out among public hospitals and other safety-net providers.

Grady and a consortium of Atlanta's nonprofit primary care clinics—again with the help of philanthropic money, nothing from the state or local governments—began researching a similar program for Atlanta in 2010. It has taken on new significance more recently since the state has refused to expand Medicaid.

Besides its outpatient clinics at the main hospital, Grady has six primary care clinics in neighborhoods around Fulton and DeKalb counties. Several other Mercy Care clinics in Atlanta serve the same population. Additionally, there are five other federally funded primary health care centers in the two counties run by nonprofit groups. It would be the first time all of these essential players have worked together.

Under the proposed plan, the primary care clinics and Grady would enroll uninsured adults in the two counties making up to 100 percent of the poverty level ($11,770 for an individual in 2015) in a Medicaid demonstration project. These are the very people caught in the so-called coverage gap—earning too much to qualify for Medicaid in nonexpansion states, but too little to be able to qualify for a subsidy to help them buy a policy through the ACA exchanges.

Each new enrollee would be assigned a "primary care medical home," meaning doctors at one of the clinics would be responsible for managing their care and would have to work with the hospital to coordinate any tests or procedures they might need. In exchange, Medicaid—like it did in Cleveland—would set a total budget for the demonstration. If it costs more to provide the services the patients need, the clinics and the hospital consortium would have to absorb the additional expenses. The state would not be at risk for any losses.

Grady plans to use the money it gets from Fulton and DeKalb for its operational expenses to provide the state's share of the cost. In the strange world of Medicaid financing, such an "intergovernmental transfer" draws many more federal dollars into the Medicaid program and would allow the state to pay essentially nothing, since Fulton and DeKalb would be the chief governmental source of funds.

The Atlanta consortium wants to target several "high cost" patient populations that drive the demand for hospital services among the poor and uninsured in the community. These include diabetes and the eye disorders related to diabetes (conditions that often result in patients going on Social Security disability when they become blind); hypertension, HIV/AIDS, and behavioral health. In similar "medical home" experiments with low-income patients around the country, the last two have been particularly costly.

Because of the way Medicaid is structured, it must be the state that seeks a waiver to conduct this experiment.

Finding Ways to Say No

But when word of the plan surfaced in early 2015, just after the general assembly had adjourned for the year, conservative legislators fumed that the waiver idea was a "back door" effort at Medicaid expansion statewide. It's not, of course, since it only would impact Fulton and DeKalb counties. (A similar consortium of safety-net providers and Memorial Hospital in Savannah also wants to try something like it.)

The legislators promised to hold hearings in the 2016 assembly session to scrutinize the proposal to make sure Georgia holds fast to its refusal to allow Medicaid expansion statewide. Predictably, in late summer of 2015, the state indicated it would not support Grady's waiver plan for even such a modest expansion of Medicaid. The cost to the state would be $3.5 million in administration—"too high," state officials said, although they did not break down how they arrived at that figure.

Again, it is a question of priorities,

This decision to turn its back on Grady's proposal comes from a state that has decided to exempt from state sales tax payments for the cost of construction material for a new domed stadium being built in downtown Atlanta for the Atlanta Falcons. It is doing the same thing for a new ballpark under construction in neighboring Cobb County for the Atlanta Braves.

The Falcons are owned by Home Depot cofounder Arthur Blank, whose net worth is thought to be around $2 billion. The Braves are owned by a division of Liberty Media, a multi-billion-dollar communications company. The justification: The new parks will secure jobs in Atlanta, and unless state and local government pony up, local political leaders fear the owners will move their teams elsewhere.

Exactly how much money will be lost because of the sales tax break has never been disclosed, but it's a good bet it is more than the $3.5 million that the state contends it can't afford to put up for Grady's Medicaid proposal.

Such is the governmental climate toward extending health care for the poor in Georgia these days. Other states, especially those in the South, have adopted a similar attitude toward public spending on the poor.

It comes with the territory, said James C. Cobb, the University of Georgia historian.

"There is a class component to public discussion of spending on health, welfare, and social programs in the South that has been around for decades now and hasn't much changed," Cobb said. "What's good for the folks who get to decide is the most important part of that equation."

In other words, unless the powerful interests that benefit most from economic development schemes and low tax rates are persuaded that more spending is needed for health care programs for the poor, there is little chance they will be enacted in the South.

Tax breaks designed to create jobs will always trump tax spending on health care and other social services, he said.

Unfortunately, the historic checkerboard of health care coverage and services for low-income Americans continues among the fifty states, some of which have made great strides with the passage of the ACA and others—like Georgia—still stuck in the bygone era of making the poor earn their keep.

Sociologist Paul Starr calls this the American "policy trap" that sets us apart from other developed nations. The United States has refused for decades to take a full and unambiguous step toward financing and implementing a system of universal health insurance the way we have for financing public schools through compulsory education.

He and others have pointed out that the middle class is greatly vested in public schools. Occasionally they even push elected officials for needed improvements and are willing to pay more in taxes to sustain quality public education. That just does not happen with spending on public health or hospitals because the real cost of health care is hidden from consumers.

As long as the United States is stuck in that policy trap, the poor will suffer the most.

You can almost hear the echo of former Georgia Governor Lester Maddox's famous quote about the deplorable condition of the state's prisons in the 1960s. Georgia's prisons would never improve unless the state "gets a better class of prisoners," Maddox predicted.

Perhaps state officials in Georgia and around the South might pay more attention to public hospitals if they started treating a better class of patients.

Going to Bat for Grady

Remember, as well, that the threat of losing federal disproportionate share money, which had been helping hospitals that took in large numbers of indigent and Medicaid patients, still exists. The Obama administration delayed the end of the program because so many states refused to expand Medicaid. But the delay is scheduled to end next year. For Grady, that would mean a loss of about $40 million annually.

And it is worth noting here that the hospital building itself is nearing fifty years of age. The $315 million renovation in the 1990s was largely new construction on the periphery; the oldest part of Grady remains and needs constant updating. Under current budget conditions, renovations can only be done in small chunks, usually one floor, one department at a time.

While metro Atlanta political leaders fall all over themselves to offer tax money for the Falcons and Braves projects, would they go to bat for Grady so that it could build a new, state-of-the-art facility like those recently opened for Parkland in Dallas and the University Medical Center in New Orleans?

Large, public hospitals like Grady Memorial in Atlanta must live in this contentious and uncertain political environment, while their competitors maneuver to find opportunities to exploit a marketplace where more Americans than ever are covered by insurance and can choose any hospital they want.

All this means that Grady must continue to rely on local philanthropic support for capital improvements and to come up with new payment and delivery methods that—short of Medicaid expansion and a renewed commitment from local government—can help offset its costs for charity care. And it must do this while at the same time recognizing that it, and likely it alone, will still be responsible for providing crisis mental health care for the poor, comprehensive services for the uninsured with HIV/AIDS and other infectious diseases, as well as emergency and acute-care treatment for immigrants who have taken up residence in our country without permission to do so.

More than a century ago, when the city and state were still trying to rebuild in the aftermath of a brutal war, Sister Mary Cecilia Carroll and three Sisters of Mercy, armed with a spirit of charity and fifty cents, set an example of public compassion for the sickly poor when they founded the city's first real hospital.

A few years later, Henry Woodfin Grady persuaded local government and business leaders that quality health care for the poor and economic development went hand in hand.

That appeal to the city and state's better angels and wiser leaders is what's gone with the wind in Georgia today. And it is not just a problem for Georgia. Clearly, the country has some unfinished business that it can ill afford to wait for another generation to complete.

Even now, as we appear to be settling down after the latest tumultuous era of health reform, it seems timely to ask: Have we reached the point where public officials, particularly those in the South, are frozen in the ice of their own indifference when it comes to the government's responsibility in caring for the poor? Can we demand a more thoughtful discussion about how to help those we have purposefully left behind?

Shouldn't we do more than help Grady and the nation's public hospitals that serve the poor to simply survive from one year to the next?

Wouldn't we be better off if our most vital hospitals are given the opportunities they deserve to thrive?

APPENDIX
WHERE ARE THE BIG PUBLIC HOSPITALS?

Defining what constitutes a public hospital is not easy. About 25 percent of the nation's 4,000 hospitals have been built with or supported by public money. And almost all of them accept payment from Medicare and Medicaid, the government-financed health insurance programs for the elderly, disabled, and medically needy.

Nor is there universal agreement on what constitutes a "safety-net" hospital, the term heard most often to describe public hospitals. Most "safety nets" are the sole provider of acute hospital care for a particular area, meaning that, without them, poor and uninsured patients would have to go outside their communities to get help.

Also, there are big differences among many of these hospitals and the large, mostly urban hospitals that were built and chartered by cities and states years ago with a specific charity mission. These larger public hospitals typically have many more indigent, uninsured, and Medicaid patients than their community hospital competitors. For a handful of them—perhaps fewer than two dozen—more than 50 percent of their patients are uninsured or on Medicaid.

Over the last two decades, many large public hospitals have become part of community-wide public health and hospital systems, like the New York City system that controls Bellevue Hospital, the nation's oldest public hospital. (There are about a dozen other hospitals in the city system.) This arrangement often allows them to share resources and offset their indigent care costs. Many of the flagship hospitals in these systems continue to carry a large burden of charity care.

There is no official list of public hospitals, but all four of the still-extant institutions this book has focused on are members of an organization called America's Essential Hospitals. Formerly known as the American Association of Public Hospitals, AEH is the nation's largest lobbying group on behalf of hospitals that provide critical services to poor and uninsured patients. A review of the full membership directory reveals the importance of major medical schools and teaching hospitals in providing this safety-net care in many states and cities. See http:// essentialhospitals.org/about-americas-essential-hospitals/ listing-of-americas-essential-hospitals-members/.

ENDNOTES

Much of the material contained in this book is the product of my many years of writing and editing stories on medicine and health care policy in both Atlanta and Louisville. The conclusions drawn in these passages are entirely mine, based on that experience, but they have been informed by more recent reporting and enhanced greatly by two outstanding books.

The first is Paul Starr's *The Social Transformation of American Medicine* (New York: Basic Books, 1982). This remains the single most comprehensive history of our nation's health care journey, and you will find numerous references to it within these pages.

The other is Martin Moran's *Atlanta's Living Legacy: A History of Grady Memorial Hospital and Its People* (Atlanta: Kimbark Publishing, 2012). Dr. Moran, a pediatrician and medical historian, has encyclopedic knowledge about Georgia's largest public hospital. I am grateful for Dr. Moran's support and encouragement in telling Grady's story in the context of what is happening with public hospitals like it across the country.

Introduction

Isobel Moutrey and her husband, Richard Beckel, agreed to a series of interviews to help illustrate how Atlanta residents who may otherwise never go to Grady come to appreciate it when they need it.

The specifics of Grady's demographics are included in the Annual Hospital Survey that all Georgia hospitals must file with the state.

The most up-to-date account of which states have adopted expansion of Medicaid can be found at the Henry K. Kaiser Family Foundation (kff.org).

Enroll America, a national coalition advocating policies to maximize coverage through the Affordable Care Act, also produces detailed mapping of where uninsured Americans live. The information is available at enrollamerica.org.

The Centers for Disease Control and Prevention (CDC) has a wide range of tools showing the prevalence of chronic disease by states and counties.

They can be accessed at cdc.gov on the Interactive Database Systems link. The Kaiser Family Foundation also provides a wealth of information about the uninsured in the United States going back over many years. The most recent reporting on this issue can be found at kff.org/uninsured.

The most interesting account of the 2012 US Supreme Court ruling on the Affordable Care Act is in Jeffrey Toobin's book, *The Oath: The Obama White House and the Supreme Court* (New York: Anchor Books, 2012).

Timothy S. Jost, of the Washington and Lee University School of Law in Lexington, Virginia, one of the nation's leading experts in health care law, discusses state challenges to the Medicaid rule in "The Tenuous Nature of the Medicaid Entitlement" (*Health Affairs* 22, no. 1 (January 2003): 145-53).

The landmark Institute of Medicine study on the risk of death and disability, called *Care without Coverage: Too Little, Too Late,* projected 20,000 Americans die each year because they lack insurance. It was published in May 2002 when an estimated 30 million Americans were without health insurance. By 2009, with the number of uninsured topping 40 million, a paper published in the *American Journal of Public Health* by the Harvard Medical School and Cambridge Health Alliance attributed 44,789 "excess deaths" due to lack of insurance.

Like the IOM study, the Harvard researchers adjusted the data for lack of education, income, and poor health habits in calculating the American death toll linked directly to being uninsured. The Harvard research also reported that Americans without insurance have a 40 percent higher risk of death than those with health insurance coverage.

Gallup surveys of Americans and the view of government responsibility for health care can be found on the company's website, gallup.com. The peak period when Americans were most likely (69 percent) to favor a larger federal role for guaranteeing health insurance came in 2007. By 2013, after the Supreme Court decision upholding the Affordable Care Act, Gallup surveys showed only 36 percent of Americans favored a large federal role. Since then, the difference has narrowed with neither side holding a majority view.

Information used in the question-and-answer sidebar in Part I, Is Charity Care a Mission or Is It the Law? comes from my own research on the subject looking at contracts public hospitals have made with local governments around the country. Larry S. Gage, a past president of the National Association of Public Hospitals (now called America's Essential Hospitals), provided a substantive account about these arrangements in a June 2012 report for the American Hospital Association's Center for Healthcare Governance.

Chapter 1: America's Cities and Their Hospitals

Besides the history lessons provided by Paul Starr and Martin Moran, background material and essential reading for this chapter can be found in the following books:

John H. Ellis. *Yellow Fever and Public Health in the New South.* Lexington, KY: University of Kentucky Press, 1981.

C. Vann Woodward. *Origins of the New South, 1877–1913.* Baton Rouge, LA: Louisiana State University Press, 1951.

Charles Rosenberg. *The Care of Strangers: The Rise of America's Hospital Systems.* New York: Basic Books, 1987.

Don H. Doyle. *New Men, New Cities, New South: Atlanta, Nashville, Charleston and Mobile, 1860–1890.* Chapel Hill, NC: University of North Carolina Press, 1990.

Franklin Garrett. *Atlanta and Environs. Volume One. A Chronicle of Its People and Events.* New York: Lewis Historical Publishing, 1954.

The portrait of Sister Mary Cecilia Carroll and the work of the Sisters of Mercy in Savannah and Atlanta are drawn from numerous historical accounts in Georgia newspapers. One of the best of these, "Neither rope ladders nor yellow fever kept Sister Cecilia Carroll from founding two hospitals," was written by volunteer archivist Rita H. DeLorme in the February 2007 of *Southern Cross,* the newspaper of the diocese of Savannah.

This book is one of the best accounts of the life of the famed newspaper editor: Harold E. Davis's *Henry Grady's New South. Atlanta: A Brave and Beautiful City* (Tuscaloosa, AL: University of Alabama Press, 1990).

The unofficial handwritten version of the resolution confirming the city of Atlanta's support for the new Grady Hospital that was set to open in 1892 is kept (along with the official document) in the Kenan Research Center at the Atlanta History Center. The handwritten version defines Grady as a "public charity," but those words have a line struck through them. They are missing from the official version.

Chapter 2: Medicine and Science

Crawford W. Long is one of the most interesting figures in Georgia history. For years his work in pioneering surgical anesthesia went unrecognized outside of a handful of physicians and surgeons who eventually found his notes and got them published. The information about Long is taken from entries about him in *The New Georgia Encyclopedia,* as well as references to him in historical accounts in surgery and anesthesiology publications.

The popular image of Civil War surgeons using whiskey as anesthesia for their wounded patients is probably more mythology than fact. Ether-based forms of anesthesia were widely in place by the end of the 1850s, according to reliable historical accounts, and it was often used in battlefield hospitals. Given the gruesomeness of their amputation tasks, many surgeons may have needed the whiskey themselves, however.

Information about the Association of American Medical Colleges is available on the group's website, aamc.org.

The 1910 *Flexner Report,* written by Abraham Flexner, set the standard for future accreditation of American medical schools. It was commissioned by the Carnegie Foundation. It was updated in 1960 and 1972, and there were numerous analyses of its impact in 2010 on the one hundredth anniversary of the landmark publication.

Information about how Emory University came to be located in Atlanta is taken from Gary S. Hauk's *A Legacy of Heart and Mind: Emory Since 1836* (Atlanta: Bookhouse, 1999).

Martin Moran's *Atlanta's Living Legacy* deals extensively with the creation of White Grady and Black Grady as well as the referenda on the city's bond issues of 1910 and 1914. These two votes are indicative of what would turn out to be decades of challenges in local financing for the public hospital.

Chapter 3: Medicine Becomes More Advanced, More Available—and Unaffordable

Much of the information in this and subsequent chapters about American medicine in the first half of the last century is derived from academic papers and several excellent histories written about the period.

In addition to Paul Starr's comparison of the difference between the European and American experience in *The Social Transformation of American Medicine,* other works include Charles Rosenberg's *The Care of Strangers: The Rise of America's Hospital System* (New York: Basic Books, 1987); Sandra Opdycke's *No One Was Turned Away: The Role of Public Hospitals in New York City since 1900* (New York: Oxford University Press, 1999); Harry F. Dowling's *City Hospitals: The Undercare of the Underprivileged* (Cambridge, MA: Harvard University Press, 1982).

Physicians for a National Health Program, which advocates for a single-payer health plan, produced an informative "Brief History: Universal Health Care Efforts in the US" that is available online at pnhp.org.

"The American Association of Labor Legislation and the Institutionalist in National Health Insurance," an article by J. Dennis Chasse, published in the *Journal of Economic Issues,* December 1994, is also an authoritative account of the effort among progressives to enact universal health care insurance.

In *The Social Transformation of American Medicine,* Paul Starr outlines how the Illinois Health Insurance Commission and other state insurance commissions began to discover that workmen's compensation plans were inadequate for coverage of hospitalization. Other studies by researchers of the American labor movement during this time make the same point.

Morris Vogel's *The Invention of the Modern Hospital: Boston, 1870–1930* (Chicago: University of Chicago Press, 1980) traces the advancement of science and the symbiotic relationship between big city hospitals and medical schools.

America's Essential Hospitals (formerly known as the National Association of Public Hospitals) has produced a history of safety-net providers that includes many of the scientific "firsts" that happened in public hospitals. The spring 2006 issue of *Safety Net* includes many of these. It and other historical reports from the group can be found at essentialhospitals.org.

The deplorable conditions at Grady were covered extensively by the *Atlanta Constitution* during this time, and articles are included in the newspaper's archives at the Atlanta History Center.

The Atlanta History Center also holds the minutes of the Grady Hospital medical staff and other hospital committees in the Grady Memorial Hospital Collection. These notes include reports of the rat infestation in 1925.

The sermon by the Reverend Leonard Broughten was covered in a June 27, 1930, *Atlanta Constitution* story.

The American Hospital Association and the Association of American Medical Colleges are both good sources for explaining how graduate medical education is paid for in the United States. The information in the Doctors in Training and How They Get Paid sidebar draws on these sources. The essay by Jacob Sunshine about resident staff pay was in a May 20, 2014, post in *Slate* magazine.

Chapter 4: The Old Ideal and the New Deal

Rosemary Stevens's *In Sickness and in Wealth: American Hospitals in the Twentieth Century* (revised edition, Baltimore: Johns Hopkins University Press, 1999) is one of the most authoritative examinations of how the hospital industry responded to the rise of health insurance and governmental social policies during this time frame. Her work, and that of Paul Starr, informs many of the conclusions I have formed in this chapter.

Southern historians, including C. Vann Woodward of Yale University, James C. Cobb of the University of Georgia, and Wayne Flynt of Auburn University, all have written extensively on the politics of New Deal programs in that region of the country.

Since 1978, the Employee Benefit Research Institute (EBRI) has been aggregating data about health insurance and other benefits offered by American employers. It also has produced numerous analytical reports about the history of health insurance in the workplace. These can be found on the group's website, ebri.org.

Rosemary Stevens's book deals extensively with the Hill–Burton hospital construction act. But the details of Georgia's unique role in securing funds from it are included in a 2013 Carnegie University paper, "Subsidies and Structure: The Lasting Impact of the Hill–Burton Program on the Hospital Industry."

Additional reporting about the financial problems besetting rural Georgia hospitals comes from various Georgia newspapers, the Georgia Hospital Association, and my own reporting on the subject for the *Atlanta Journal-Constitution* and, more recently, for this book. It should be noted that the plight of America's rural hospitals is in many ways similar to that of large, urban hospitals, especially as it relates to their dependence on Medicare and Medicaid payment for survival. Addressing the issues specifically connected to rural hospitals, however, will require reorganizing how health care is delivered in sparsely populated areas. Telemedicine, better coordination of care with federally funded primary care clinics, more use of physician assistants and certified nurse practitioners, and establishing urgent care outposts with emergency medical technicians and better emergency transport capability may replace the need for some rural hospitals.

Chapter 5: Race, Medicare, and Medicaid

In 2015, the nation marked the fiftieth anniversary of the enactment of Medicare and Medicaid. The year before, we celebrated the fiftieth anniversary of the Civil Rights Act, the pillars of President Lyndon Johnson's Great Society programs. Hundreds of articles in the mainstream press and in social and medical journals recounted the historic impact of these landmark laws. *Health Affairs*, the nation's leading journal on health policy, has followed developments in Medicare and especially Medicaid quite extensively. The conclusions in this chapter are drawn from the work published there and in other respected publications.

Additionally, two books are important to this chapter. Jonathan Engel's *Poor People's Medicine: Medicaid and Charity Care since 1965* (Durham, NC: Duke University Press, 2006) examines the underpinnings of the nation's health insurance program for the poor. Jerry Gentry's *Grady Baby: A Year in the Life of Atlanta's Grady Hospital* (Jackson, MS: University Press of Mississippi, 1999) provides the deepest and most fascinating dive into the desegregation of the hospital. Gentry's book is mostly about a year in the life of the patients, physicians, and staff at the hospital's obstetrics clinic. But his account of how "the Gradys" came to an end after the passage of Medicare is no doubt similar to what happened in many public hospitals in the South during the civil rights era.

There are conflicting accounts of how the Centers for Disease Control and Prevention came to be located in Atlanta, but they all agree on the key player being Coca-Cola president Robert W. Woodruff and his interest in connecting the Emory University School of Medicine to the study of malaria and other communicable diseases. The information for this recounting comes from news interviews with Randy Gue, curator of the modern political and historical collections at Emory's Robert W. Woodruff Library.

As a reporter in Atlanta in the late 1980s, I covered the, at times, contentious negotiations between the Morehouse School of Medicine and Emory University School of Medicine to jointly staff Grady. The two schools renewed their agreement on Grady staffing in 2013.

How Medicare claims came to be administered at the state level is documented by Paul Starr, Rosemary Stevens, and others.

The impact of Medicare on the life-span of Americans is taken from a series of reports on the Commonwealth Fund website entitled *Medicare at 50 Years*, commonwealthfund.org.

According to several historical accounts, the term *three-layer cake*, which was used to describe the proposed plan to cover hospital care for the elderly, physician care for the elderly, and medical care in general for the poor, was first coined by House Ways and Means Committee Chairman Wilbur Mills of Ohio in his discussion with President Johnson during the run up to the passage of Medicare. The plan for the poor, originally envisioned as Medicare's Part C, never materialized, and the three-layer cake never got baked. Instead, a separate program for the poor called Medicaid, to be shared with the states, was enacted outside of the Medicare program.

More information on the "dual eligible" issue of elderly and disabled people on both Medicare and Medicaid can be found through the Kaiser Commission on Medicaid and the Uninsured on the Kaiser Family Foundation website, kff.org.

Chapter 6: Getting to Now

Paul Starr's most recent book on health care, *Remedy and Reaction: The Peculiar American Struggle over Health Care Reform* (New Haven, CT: Yale University Press, 2011) picks up where *Social Transformation of American Medicine* left off. As an advisor to First Lady Hillary Clinton during the failed effort at reform during the Bill Clinton era, Starr had a unique perspective on the politics of enacting a more comprehensive approach to the issue. He addresses them in *Remedy and Reaction* and examines other reform efforts leading up to the enactment of the Affordable Care Act of 2010. Others, including presidential biographers, have tackled the same issues during this period, but mostly as a question of politics. These accounts are also important to the understanding of how, with the election of Barack Obama in 2008, the nation seemed finally ready to take a big step toward universal coverage.

As outlined in previous chapter notes, there is a wealth of information about the insurance status of Americans that goes back decades. The data sources for this information can be found in the reports of the Employee Benefit Research Institute, which has thoroughly documented health insurance benefits provided by employers, and the Commonwealth Fund and the Kaiser Family Foundation. The Kaiser Commission on Medicaid and the Uninsured is a rich source for data on Medicaid enrollment. (The data included in this chapter are largely drawn from the Kaiser Commission.)

All these groups rely on independent surveys as well as updated Census Bureau data. The data may at times seem to conflict, but closer examination usually reveals the difference is in the specific survey being examined for analysis. Some surveys, for instance, exclude Medicare-eligible respondents. Others adjust for newly employed respondents who are temporarily not covered by a plan while they wait to become eligible for their new employer plan. Others account for these same people as having been uninsured at some point during the survey year. It is always advisable to closely examine any survey from which data are drawn.

The oft-repeated claim that Obamacare amounts to a "government takeover of health care," was awarded *Politifact's* Lie of the Year in 2010. Despite the dubious honor, the claim continues to resonate with many Americans.

As noted in the Introduction, Gallup polling on the role the federal government should play in health care flip-flopped between 2007 and 2014. These polls can be found at gallup.com.

The Centers for Medicare & Medicaid Services provides an explanation for how the disproportionate share hospital program works at CMS.gov.

Florida's newspapers and an independent, nonprofit source of health care news in the state, *Health News Florida*, extensively covered the story of Governor Rick Scott's flip-flop on Medicaid expansion. The account here is drawn from that coverage.

Another nonprofit news source, *Georgia Health News* (georgiahealthnews. com), as well as the *Atlanta Journal-Constitution,* have covered the state's opposition to Medicaid expansion thoroughly in recent years. I have also paid attention to and written about the issue as well.

The Georgia Budget and Policy Institute, the best source of information on state spending on health, education, and welfare programs, provided the financial analysis for why the state should expand Medicaid, cited in this chapter. The GBPI estimates the actual cost of expansion to the state to be around $200 million per year, or $2.1 billion over the first ten years.

The economic impact of Medicaid expansion in Georgia referenced in this chapter was compiled by William S. Custer of the Institute of Health Administration, Georgia State University. Custer's numbers on cost to the state mirror those of the GBPI. The state, on the other hand, projects the cost of Medicaid expansion at more than twice that amount, $4.5 billion over ten years, but it has never provided a substantive breakdown at how it arrived at that figure.

Wayne Flynt, professor emeritus at Auburn University, has been a longtime source of thoughtful commentary on social, health, and education programs in Alabama and the rest of the South. He is a prolific author as well. His comments in this chapter about the connection between the health of children and school performance were included in a January 2014 piece he wrote for AL.com, the website for several Alabama newspapers.

Information used to report Nursing Homes and Their Clout in Georgia comes from my own reporting as well as that of *Georgia Health News* and the *Atlanta Journal-Constitution,* both of which have written extensively on the subject. The newspaper has closely examined the campaign contributions to Georgia's elected officials from nursing home owners and their family members as well as campaign funds provided by the hospital and insurance industry in the state.

Chapter 7: Bridging the Gap between the Races

Interviews with Tracie Steadman, the stroke patient, and Dr. Raul Nogueira, who removed the clot from her brain, were conducted in the neuroscience department at Grady Hospital. Tracie now works at the hospital as a patient navigator and is covered by the hospital's health insurance plan.

Data documenting the morbidity and mortality of the health care system in the United States versus health systems in other industrialized nations is widely available through the World Health Organization, the CDC, and the Commonwealth Fund, among other sources. These data should always be examined for subtle differences in time studied, population estimates, and cost distinctions, all of which can affect rankings of individual countries. T. R. Reid's *The Healing of America: A Global Quest for Better, Cheaper, and Fairer Health Care* (New York: Penguin Books. 2010) is one of the best books written on the subject.

Numerous studies document the health disparities between the races and income levels of Americans. Over the last thirty years, this is an area rich in research within the public health community. Former Surgeon General David Satcher, now director of the Satcher Health Leadership Institute at the Morehouse School of Medicine, heads a group of national researchers who report regularly on health disparities. The CDC releases a periodic

Health Disparities and Inequalities Report, the latest of which is available at cdc.gov. The American Heart Association, the American Cancer Society, and other advocacy groups for prevention and treatment of chronic diseases also report yearly statistics that usually include comparisons of mortality and disease incidence rates among the races.

President George W. Bush's comments about how poor Americans can get access to health care by going to hospital emergency rooms were made in Cleveland in July 2007 and widely covered by the press. His comments were in response to his threat to veto the expansion of the Children's Health Insurance Program that was working its way through Congress at the time. He made good on his threat. President Barack Obama signed an expansion order for the program after Democrats took over the House and Senate in 2009.

There are several references in this chapter to the Avon Foundation for Women study published in 2014 that was the first to estimate a yearly death toll caused by the disparity in treatment of low-income black women with breast cancer compared to white women in the most populous American cities. The study can be found on the foundation website, avonfoundation.org.

One of the most interesting analyses of how Medicaid eligibility changed the delivery and cost of caring for low-income pregnant women and their babies was written in 1996 and published in the *Journal of Political Economy*. It was coauthored by Jonathan Gruber, a Massachusetts Institute of Technology economics professor who later was used as a consultant by the Obama White House to project the cost of the Affordable Care Act. (It was Gruber who infamously declared that the act was passed, at least in part, because of the "stupidity of the American voter," making him a favorite target of the law's critics.)

Former Vice President Dick Cheney, at the age of seventy-one, received a heart transplant in March of 2012 after using a left ventricular assist device (LVAD), which assists the diseased heart, for about twenty months.

The first indication of the high cost of Grady's outpatient kidney dialysis unit was included in a report about potential cost savings to the hospital foundation and the Fulton-DeKalb Hospital Authority by Alvarez & Marsal Healthcare Industry Group in 2007. At the time, as an editorial writer for the *Atlanta Journal-Constitution*, I wrote about it and called on hospital authorities to confront the issue rather than ignore it. The clinic remained open until the new governing body took control of the hospital in 2009.

The *New York Times* Atlanta-based reporter Kevin Sack provided detailed coverage of the plight of undocumented immigrants with kidney disease who could no longer get outpatient dialysis at Grady after the unit closed in 2009. Reporters for the *Atlanta Journal-Constitution* also thoroughly covered the controversial closing of the clinic.

The study of Georgia dialysis facilities and the referral rates for transplant patients with end-stage renal disease was published in the *Journal of the American Medical Association* in August 2015. It was researched and written by Rachel Patzer of the Emory University School of Medicine and Rollins School of Public Health.

The Centers for Medicare & Medicaid Services provides a history and overview of the End Stage Renal Disease Program on its website. It also includes detailed information about the cost of the program over the years. Other researchers have studied the impact the ESRD program has had on Medicare costs, changes in how services are paid for, and the rise of for-profit clinics that have resulted from enacting the program. One of the best papers on these and other issues related to ESRD was published in a September 2012 issue of *Health Affairs*. The lead author of the study was Brown University researcher Shailender Swaminathan.

Dr. Sheryl Gabram agreed to a series of interviews about her work at the Georgia Cancer Center for Excellence at Grady. She also provided some of the research and statistical data used in the cancer disparities section of this chapter, including the "Time to Treatment" study published in *The Breast Journal* in 2011.

The study about how often breast cancer patients are recommended for gene expression profiling in regions of the country where there is a wide disparity in income was published in *Health Affairs* in April 2015.

Dr. Otis W. Brawley of the American Cancer Society has been a very helpful source of information on cancer and public policy since his days at Grady.

Chapter 8: On the Front Lines of AIDS, Funding Remains Uncertain

I spoke with several patients and staff members of Grady's Infectious Disease Program (IDP) for the personal anecdotes used in this chapter. The young patients agreed to discuss their stories as long as they were not identified in any way. Jonathan, the patient discussed at the start of the chapter, chose that name for his story. As of 2015, he continues to do well on his HIV treatment plan and visits the Grady clinic regularly.

The best source for the incidence rate, mortality, and new HIV infections in the United States remains the Atlanta-based CDC. The agency, in coordination with state and public health departments around the country, releases new data continuously in an effort to monitor trends in the epidemic. At a deeper level, the CDC also periodically analyzes five- and ten-year trend lines. Other organizations also use these studies to tease out specific data within geographic areas and population groups, an exercise which takes longer and results in reports that may seem out of date at times. But these deeper dives into the data can be very helpful in confirming more recent anecdotal evidence about how the epidemic is evolving.

Emory University researchers reported the increased risk of gay black men contracting HIV compared to gay white men at a 2014 Conference on Retroviruses and Opportunistic Infections in Atlanta. The ongoing research is called the Involve(men)t Study. More information about the study can be found at prismhealth.us.

Carl Schmid, deputy executive director of the AIDS Institute, has commented in numerous news reports that some policies sold in the first year of the ACA inadequately covered drug costs for HIV patients. Kathye Gorosh of the AIDS Foundation of Chicago made these comments to me in an interview in August 2014. In mid-2015, CMS made an attempt to deal with some of these pricing issues in the plans being sold for 2016. CMS warned insurers not to place all or most drugs used to treat specific conditions in their highest tier, requiring patients who need them to pay significant out-of-pocket costs.

The study of new infections in Southern states is taken from a 2012 paper by the Southern HIV/AIDS Strategy Initiative (SASI), an arm of the Duke

Center for Health Policy and Inequalities Research, Duke University. SASI issues regular updates analyzing CDC data on HIV within Southern states.

The Kaiser Family Foundation reported the HIV testing data in a June 2015 fact sheet on the foundation's website, kff.org.

Information about the cost of drugs for patients with HIV and other sexually transmitted diseases comes from patient advocacy groups in Georgia, Illinois, and Florida, which have monitored the drug benefit programs made available to the newly insured through the Affordable Care Act state exchanges. Because the plans available on the exchanges can alter each year what drugs are covered and how much insurance will pay for them, it will be important for these groups and the patients they help to stay up-to-date on costs and benefits. The continuing high cost of prescription drugs, even those that are available as generics, has turned out to be one of the largest drivers of increased insurance rates since the ACA was fully enacted.

Information about the Ryan White HIV/AIDS Program is available through the Health Resources Services Administration, an arm of the US Department of Health and Human Services. The act is named after the Indiana teenager who fought AIDS-related discrimination after he was expelled from a public school when diagnosed with AIDS at the age of thirteen. He died in 1990 at nineteen years of age. The Ryan White Fund has, for years, been the largest federal grant program for education, services, and treatment of low-income and uninsured Americans with HIV.

The role public hospitals have played in providing the first line of defense in the treatment of HIV/AIDS has been addressed in several books and medical publications. Information about the HIV programs at Grady, Cook County Hospital in Chicago, and Jackson Memorial Hospital in Miami came from interviews with officials of HIV clinics and advocates in those cities.

Dr. David Reznik, chief of dental services and Oral Health Center director at the Grady IDP, is one of Atlanta's leading HIV/AIDS advocates. He agreed to several interviews over the course of research for this chapter, including details on how he came to create the oral health program for HIV patients in Atlanta.

Chapter 9: Mental Health: The Continuing Crisis in Caring for the Poor

The Grady Hospital Assertive Community Treatment teams allowed me to attend one of their daily meetings, provided I protected the identities of their patients. The names of the patients referred to at the beginning of this chapter are not their real names.

My reporting on mental health policy issues goes back to 1983 at the *Courier-Journal* in Louisville, Kentucky. A colleague Bob Pierce and I examined the impact of deinstitutionalization of Kentucky's mental hospitals and the lack of follow-up care for the chronically mentally ill in the community. It was in that reporting when I first discovered the efficacy of the Assertive Community Treatment team approach being employed in Dane County, Wisconsin.

On a personal note, I must add that it is profoundly sad that this approach, more than thirty years later, is still not widely used around the country. The use of coordinated teams of doctors, nurses, and social workers in the treatment of low-income people with chronic disease holds great promise as has been shown by the success of these teams working with the mentally ill and similarly successful approaches in assuring prenatal care for low-income pregnant women.

The quality-of-care issues inside Georgia's state mental hospitals came to light through the excellent reporting of Andy Miller and Alan Judd in the *Atlanta Journal-Constitution*. The newspaper's reporting eventually led to a federal lawsuit filed against the state to close some of the hospitals and improve staffing at others. As of mid-2015, the state remained under court order to carry out terms of a settlement agreement in the suit.

E. Fuller Torrey's *Nowhere to Go: The Tragic Odyssey of the Homeless Mentally Ill* (New York: Harper Collins, 1989) is one of the best accounts of the nation's failure to care for the chronically mentally ill homeless population. Fuller, who has written numerous books on the subject, is founder of the Treatment Advocacy Center in Arlington, Virginia. The advocacy center also provided information about the level of state funding for mental illness used in this chapter.

The American Mental Health Counselors Association produced a report in April 2015 on the problems with access to mentally ill patients in states that have not expanded Medicaid. The report is available through the group's website at amhca.org.

Thresholds, a Chicago-based advocacy group for the mentally ill, produced a November 2013 policy brief outlining the cost effectiveness of community-based treatment, such as that provided by ACT teams, compared to the cost of institutional care and nursing home placement for behavioral health patients.

Grady Hospital provided the statistics about the increasing demand on its behavioral health unit since the close of several state mental institutions.

Richard G. Frank's article, "Be Careful What You Ask For," examining the role of Medicaid in the nation's mental health funding, was published in *Health Affairs* in June 2003. Frank was then a professor of health economics at Harvard Medical School and a leading expert on mental health care funding. Now on leave from Harvard, Frank was appointed assistant secretary for planning and evaluation in the Department of Health and Human Services in March 2014.

The information about the staggering numbers of mentally ill inmates in local jails and state prisons are taken from US Department of Justice, Bureau of Justice Statistics.

The coordinated approach among law enforcement, court officials, and mental health providers taken in San Antonio was reported extensively by *Kaiser Health News* in 2014.

The National Health Care for the Homeless Council produced an important policy paper about the potential impact of Medicaid expansion among the prison and jail population in January 2013. It is available on the group's website, nhchc.org. The study includes data about the inmates in Washington state who would qualify for Medicaid if it were to take advantage of the Medicaid expansion under the ACA. Washington enacted expansion later that year.

Chapter 10: Trauma Care: The Service We Take for Granted

The trauma cases of Richard Beckel and Sylvia Ennis and their trauma surgeon, Dr. Omar Danner, came to my attention while interviewing Dr. Danner about his trauma work at Grady Memorial Hospital. Isobel Moutrey, Beckel's wife, talked at length about her husband's long stay at Grady as well as her own experiences there while he recovered. I first met Sylvia Ennis at a ceremony honoring the DeKalb County emergency medical technicians who stabilized her and brought her into the Grady trauma unit. Neither Beckel nor Ennis had been to Grady before sustaining their severe injuries. Nor had Moutrey, so they provided a unique perspective on the place. All three are now public advocates for Georgia's largest public hospital.

Dr. Thomas M. Scalea, physician in chief at Maryland Shock Trauma Hospital, provided much of the information about trauma care in recent years at American hospitals. He is an expert in the field. In my early years at the *Atlanta Journal-Constitution*, I covered the growth and decline of Georgia's trauma network and became familiar with the policy and financial issues connected to the field.

The American College of Surgeons is the professional group that monitors quality control at the nation's trauma hospitals. It also produces regular reports on the death and disabilities connected to the lack of or poorly coordinated trauma care. The CDC also keeps data on the impact of trauma around the country. Data from both of these sources are included in this chapter.

Grady Hospital provided the data on its trauma center.

The first reporting on the new competition in trauma services came from news organizations in Texas and Florida, where the Hospital Corporation of America began applying for trauma designation for several of its suburban community hospitals. *Kaiser Health News* and *Health News Florida* have also covered the Florida controversy. The *Tampa Bay Times* has produced the most exhaustive coverage of the issue, including being the first to report the existence of high trauma activation fees at Florida's HCA hospitals that had received trauma status from the state.

Connie Porter's *Tampa Bay Times* opinion piece about how she felt the trauma fees were being abused in Florida forms the basis for the sidebar A

$30,000 Fee to Go to a Trauma Center? How'd That Happen?

The Georgia Trauma Task Force provided the data about the impact of trauma costs on Georgia hospitals. The task force was created to support a statewide referendum in 2010 to levy a $10 yearly fee on motor vehicle tags that could have been used to offset the high cost of trauma centers. The referendum was soundly defeated, however.

The impact of Florida's trauma expansion of the Ryder Trauma Center in Miami comes from interviews with hospital officials at Jackson Memorial Hospital. The numbers have also been reported by local news organizations in the Miami area.

Chapter 11: Orphans

A visit to the crumbling shells of Charity Hospital in New Orleans and the old Cook County Hospital in Chicago brings a tinge of sadness to anyone who dares stand in their shadows, as I have in recent years. They were the very definition of public hospitals during an era when public administration took a back seat to the mission of care for the poor. Both hospitals could boast of scientific and clinical care advancements. But they also were bastions of political patronage where patient care was, at times, woefully inadequate and no one seemed to care. There have been numerous books and news stories written about their histories, accomplishments, and shortcomings. I have mined many of these for use in this chapter, but two stand out:

The best explanation about Charity Hospital's closing after Hurricane Katrina comes from an article, "Why Was New Orleans Charity Hospital Allowed to Die," by Roberta Brandes Gratz in the April 27, 2011, edition of *The Nation*. Gratz's reporting traces the plan behind closing Charity even though it could have reopened after the storm, and the disruption that caused to the city's large population of poor and uninsured residents who relied on Charity. In 2015, on the tenth anniversary of Katrina, other news organizations returned to New Orleans to tell Charity's story, repeating much of the reporting that originated with Gratz. These more recent updates came just at the time the state was opening the new University Medical Center, designed to handle many of Charity's former patients with state-of-the-art acute-care facilities and a new network of outpatient clinics.

David A. Ansell's *County: Life, Death and Politics at Chicago's Public Hospital*
(Chicago: Academy Chicago Publishers, 2011) dwells on the old hospital's
last years of life. Ansell was a resident physician at County and instrumental
in securing better patient care during the 1970s and 1980s, a tumultuous
period highlighted by conflicts among the medical staff, hospital administrators, and government officials. He eventually became a member of the
county board that governed County, which closed in 2002 to make way for
the new John H. Stroger, Jr. Hospital of Cook County. He is now vice president of clinical affairs and chief medical director of Rush University Medical
Center, just down the street from the old County Hospital.

The interview with patient Richard Romanowski at the end of the chapter
was broadcast by Chicago public television station WTTW, Jan. 29, 2014.
Romanowski is a patient at the Erie Family Health Center, which, along
with County Hospital is a part of a Cook County consortium that provides primary and acute care to newly eligible Medicaid patients.

The US Census Bureau's designation of the South and other regions of
the country are outlined on the bureau's website. The definition of the
"Old South" used in the South and Medicaid sidebar in this chapter is
the one generally accepted by historians to mean the states that were part
of the Confederacy at the time of the Civil War. The information about
which states have expanded Medicaid under terms of the Affordable
Care Act is taken from the Kaiser Family Foundation, which keeps close
track of the issue.

Chapter 12: Hope and Reality

During the height of the Grady Hospital crisis in 2007 and 2008, as
an editorial board member for the *Atlanta Journal-Constitution,* I wrote
a series of "Saving Grady" editorials and columns—forty-six different
pieces—outlining the problems and potential solutions to address governance issues at the hospital. Reporters Andy Miller, Gayle White, and the
news staff of the paper provided extensive coverage of developments at
Grady. Business leaders in Atlanta credit news coverage of Grady during
this time as a contributing factor for switching control of day-to-day operations at the hospital from the Fulton-DeKalb Hospital Authority to a
nonprofit, community-based governing board.

Sam A. Williams's book, *The CEO as Urban Statesman* (Macon, GA: Mercer University Press, 2014), includes a chapter on the Atlanta business community's involvement in the Grady changeover. Williams is the former president of the Metro Atlanta Chamber of Commerce.

Information about the Mercy Care clinics and their mission in Atlanta is available online at mercyatlanta.org. Tom Andrews, president of the group, provided additional background for this chapter.

The late Richard Whitt, a Pulitzer Prize–winning investigative reporter, revealed the cost overruns and minority contracting problems in the *Atlanta Journal-Constitution* in 1995 during the Grady renovation project.

In May 9, 2007 and June 27, 2007 opinion pieces, *Atlanta Journal-Constitution* Editorial Page Editor Cynthia Tucker criticized then Gov. Sonny Perdue and state Republican leaders for not being interested in providing state financial assistance to save Grady. She characterized Perdue's attitudes about Atlanta as ranging "from hostility to indifference."

I examined Fulton County budgets going back over a period of thirty years to determine that funding for Grady operations that comes from the state's largest county has not kept pace with the growth in the hospital's operating budget or the increase in indigent patients it serves.

Unfortunately, public interest in improving the quality of care at American public hospitals often doesn't show up until after horror stories come to light through local news coverage. That was the case in both the Los Angeles and Dallas cases referenced in this chapter. The *Los Angeles Times* blew the whistle on serious problems with patient care at the Martin Luther King/Charles Drew Medical Center in the Watts section of the city. The *Dallas Morning News* provided extensive coverage of problems at Parkland Memorial Hospital, including the insightful analysis of the relationship between the hospital and the University of Texas Southwestern Medical School.

Major news organizations in Florida, including the *Miami Herald, Tampa Bay Times,* and *Health News Florida* covered the 2012 legislation that required public hospitals to explore the benefits of selling or leasing their facilities to for-profit or nonprofit hospital corporations. The report prepared for Jackson Memorial Hospital in Miami was produced by Public

Fiscal Management, Inc., of Orlando. It contains very useful information comparing Jackson to other Florida hospitals, as well as Grady, Parkland, Cook County, and several other large "benchmark" public hospitals around the country. The report is available on the Jackson Memorial website, jacksonhealth.org.

The figure of 1,170 yearly deaths that could be attributed to Georgia's refusal to expand Medicaid comes from the Center for American Progress, a progressive think tank based in Washington. The center's staff extrapolated data from a September 2012 study in the *New England Journal of Medicine* that concluded there was a reduced risk of mortality for low-income patients in three states that had expanded Medicaid when compared to neighboring states that had not after the ACA was enacted. The *NEJM* study found that low-income elderly, nonwhite, and rural residents of the expansion states were most likely to benefit from becoming eligible for Medicaid. The *NEJM* study was conducted by researchers at the Harvard School of Public Health.

The dollar figures and job-creation projections connected to the expansion of the Savannah River port project and the tax breaks provided to television and movie production companies working in Georgia were taken from news stories as well as state economic development press releases and promotions.

The picture of Grady's financial health was last updated in August 2015. It was confirmed by CEO John Haupert and board chairman Pete Correll. The hospital's fiscal year closes December 31 each year, and it files an annual cost report for the purposes of Medicare reimbursement with the Centers for Medicare & Medicaid Services the following year.

The information about MetroHealth in Cleveland and the comparisons with Grady's plan for a similar program to enroll low-income adults under a Medicaid waiver comes from my own reporting on both projects. The Grady plan was outlined to me in August 2015 by hospital administrators and officials of a consortium of Atlanta's primary care safety-net providers. More information about the Cleveland program can be found in an article entitled "MetroHealth Care Plus: Effects of a Prepared Safety Net on Quality of Care in a Medicaid Expansion Population" by Case Western Reserve University researchers in the July 2015 edition of *Health Affairs*.

It's difficult to determine how state officials in Georgia arrive at some of the projections they have made about the cost of Medicaid expansion. Still, these projections are routinely touted as a reason for why the state cannot afford it and rarely are questioned, except by advocates for expansion. For instance, the state has not provided a breakdown of what it claims will be $3.5 million in yearly "costs" to administer the Medicaid waiver Grady is seeking. That amount seems greatly inflated since Grady will absorb most of the cost of administration of the program through the current subsidy it gets from Fulton and DeKalb counties. The state would only need to pass along the required paperwork to Washington to keep the program going. Grady and the primary care providers participating in the program would be liable for any potential losses, not the state.

The state's lack of transparency on this funding issue is similar to its claim that Medicaid expansion overall will cost Georgia taxpayers $4.5 billion over ten years. That figure is more than double the projections that the Georgia State University cost-benefit analysis referenced in chapter 6 shows. But without more details from the state, it is impossible to say which projections are most accurate.

The cost and public financing connected to building a new domed stadium for the Atlanta Falcons and a new park for the Atlanta Braves has been covered extensively in the *Atlanta Journal-Constitution* and other Atlanta news organizations.

James C. Cobb is professor of history at the University of Georgia and author of numerous books about Southern politics and culture. His most recent book, *The South and America since World War II*, was published by Oxford University Press in 2010. In an interview, he provided great context for how and why public officials in the South prioritize state spending, as well as how they react to being forced into partnerships with the federal government in funding programs for the poor.

In August 2011, a year after the ACA was enacted but before the US Supreme Court ruled that Medicaid expansion was voluntary for the states, the Republican Governor's Association issued a sixteen-page report on alternatives to Medicaid. The recommendations included in that report form the basis for the sidebar Republican Alternatives to Medicaid that is examined in this chapter.

INDEX

ACKNOWLEDGMENTS

I always believed that if you are a newspaper reporter in a big city and you can't find enough good stories at a public hospital to fill up a book, you should seriously think about getting out of the business.

But the truth is I had to get out of the business before I finally had time to write a whole book about what makes public hospitals so interesting…and newsworthy.

The journalistic pull of Grady Memorial Hospital was one of the reasons I uprooted my family from Louisville to Atlanta nearly thirty years ago. As a science and medicine writer, metro editor, and editorial board member at the *Atlanta Journal-Constitution,* I came to understand and deeply appreciate Grady's public health importance—as well as its critical shortcomings. I long ago stopped counting all the stories I wrote, or edited, about Grady.

The original peg for this book was the 2010 passage of the Patient Protection and Affordable Care Act, the most significant health care law since Medicare was enacted a half century ago. I wanted to get some sense of how public hospitals, which have long been the safety net for the poor, were about to change now that the country was moving toward universal access to insurance.

But the tone of political rhetoric and the rancor of the opposition to the ACA highlighted the organized obstruction to it at the state level in Georgia, turning my research—and ultimately the book—in a different direction. Once again, America was confronting its decades-old resistance toward joining the rest of the industrialized world in guaranteeing access to health care for all its citizens. And once again, these hospitals were being called upon to care for those we purposely have left behind.

I am indebted to the hundreds of academic experts, physicians, and other journalists who have studied the history of American health care and hospitals over the years. My bookshelf, and computer hard drive, is overflowing with important research and analysis that helped me carve out a book about the unique role of public hospitals in the nation's health care reform journey.

My work in Atlanta has been helped by the cooperation of the public affairs staff at Grady, especially Denise Simpson, the long-time hospital spokesperson who seems to live there. My standing arrangement with Denise and her bosses at Grady was that she would help arrange interviews with doctors and patients when I was inside the hospital, but I was free to deal with them directly when they were away from the hospital. The hospital did not exercise any editorial control or pre-publication review of the manuscript.

Grady CEO John Haupert, as well as the CEOs of several other major public hospitals around the country, provided context for what I was finding in my research. I appreciated these frank discussions.

The staff at the James G. Kenan Research Center at the Atlanta History Center was helpful in finding the 1890s ordinances and documents that established Grady as the city's first public hospital. The history center was a treasure trove for much more, including early photos and newspaper coverage of the hospital in the years preceding digital archiving. The best reference librarian I know, and my good friend, Dorothy Shea, helped me retrieve more recent coverage of public hospital controversies from the digital archives of a dozen or so major American newspapers.

My editor, Ron Sauder, who also is publisher of Secant Publishing, has been with me almost from the beginning of this project. As a former communications executive at Emory University, Ron was aware of my reporting about Grady. His familiarity with the Atlanta health care marketplace and his connections to graduate medical education programs and academic medical centers around the country were invaluable. Sandra Wendel, who copyedited the manuscript, is a gift to writers who, like me, are concentrating on the big picture and sometimes missing the important detail. Thanks, Sandra, for cleaning up my messy sentences and finding the holes and contradictions in the manuscript that I missed.

A special note of thanks goes to Katie and Patrick King, who put up with their father staying late at work for their entire childhood. They, and their late mother, Anne Harbison King, understood the life of a journalist and made it easy for me to be a husband and father at the same time. They mean more to me than any byline, including the one on the front cover. I love you guys. And to Erin Walls McFall, the best stepdaughter a man could ever have, thank you for the encouragement and support. Thanks as well to Erin, Katie, Patrick and their friends for touting the book on Facebook and other social media.

Lastly, my wife Sherry was the first to suggest there was a book inside me waiting to be written. She graciously tolerated my dominance of our front "office" while I was online researching and on the phone conducting interviews. More important, however, was her steadfast support for finishing the book last year when she was recovering from breast cancer.

As a surgery patient at Grady, Sherry experienced firsthand the challenge of navigating through a public hospital chartered to care for the poor. For example, during an overnight stay at Grady, the breast cancer patient with whom Sherry shared a room spent the entire night on the telephone trying to find a relative or friend who could take her home to recover and help her get the follow-up care she would need. Hopefully, Grady did not lose track of her after surgery. This one patient's plight made it clearer than ever why I needed to write about public hospitals.

In the hard days of chemotherapy and radiation treatment that followed for Sherry after her surgery, we both understood how lucky we are to have friends and family who helped us deal with cancer and make it through the final research and writing of this book.

We did it, didn't we? Thank you, Sweet Shereen.

Mike King
Atlanta, 2016

ABOUT THE AUTHOR

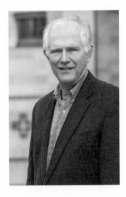

For nearly four decades Mike King worked as a reporter, Washington correspondent, science and medicine editor, and opinion writer for the *Courier-Journal* in Louisville, Kentucky, and the *Atlanta Journal-Constitution*. He and his wife live in Atlanta.